Ultrasonography in Obstetrics and Gynecology

Ultrasonography in Obstetrics and Gynecology

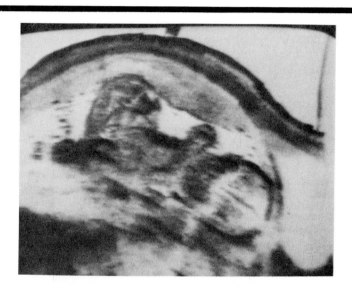

John C. Hobbins
Fred Winsberg

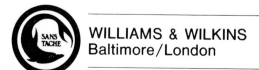 **WILLIAMS & WILKINS**
Baltimore/London

Made in the United States of America

Reprinted March 1978
Reprinted June 1978
Reprinted July 1979
Reprinted January 1980

Library of Congress Cataloging in Publication Data
Hobbins, John C.
    Obstetrical ultrasound.

    (Ultrasonography in obstetrics and gynecology)
    Includes indexes.
    1. Ultrasonics in obstetrics. I. Winsberg, Fred, joint author. II. Title. III. Series.
[DNLM: 1. Ultrasonics—Diagnostic use. 2. Obstetrics. 3. Gynecologic diseases—Diagnosis. WQ100 H682u]
RG527.5.U48H6   618.2′07′54   77-8195
ISBN 0-683-04088-X

Composed and printed at the
Waverly Press, Inc.
Mt. Royal and Guilford Aves.
Baltimore, Md. 21202, U.S.A.

Preface

The applications of ultrasound are expanding as more medical subspecialties use the modality and as manufacturers provide more sophisticated instruments. In fact, it is increasingly difficult to cover all facets of ultrasound in one text, and books have begun to emerge which address themselves to more specific subjects such as echocardiography, ophthalmological ultrasound, etc. In particular, the field of obstetrical ultrasound has burgeoned over the past 5 years simply because ultrasound as a non-invasive diagnostic tool has a wide variety of practical applications which are extremely useful in obstetrical practice.

It is interesting that both radiologist and obstetrician are examining the obstetrical patient with ultrasound. Since the radiologist has expertise in all forms of imagery and the obstetrician is trained to apply basic physiology to information obtained from any test, each could benefit from the experience of the other by working together. Yet, in most instances, this is not the case. Although some obstetricians now have ultrasound units in their office, in the majority of hospitals the patient is referred to the radiologist with a succinct request, "? maturity." In interpreting the technician's scan, the radiologist is without knowledge of the intricacies of the patient's condition; and the obstetrician, who could benefit from subtle information displayed on the ultrasound screen, is left with a biparietal diameter reading and a two-word description of placental location.

This text is a concerted effort by a radiologist and an obstetrician to digest the available literature, coordinate it with original data and many years of combined experience in obstetrical ultrasound, and to present the condensed product in an easily extractable form. No chapter is written exclusively by one author, and each concept has been treated so that ultrasonic findings are correlated with basic principles in fetal and maternal physiology.

In any new field many controversial issues emerge simply because insufficient data are available to prove or disprove an initial concept or hypothesis. In dealing with controversial matters, we have elected to take a stand by injecting our common opinion based on our observation in an effort to provide the reader with a uniform approach to difficult subjects. It will be quite clear where these opinions appear.

This book is directed to any member of the health profession who participates in the care of the obstetrical and gynecological patient. Our aim is to initiate the uninitiated and to further inform the already informed.

John C. Hobbins, M.D.
Associate Professor
of Obstetrics and Gynecology
and Diagnostic Radiology
Yale University School of Medicine

Director of Obstetrics
and Special Maternal Care
Yale New Haven Hospital

Fred Winsberg, M.D.
Associate Professor
of Radiology
McGill University, Faculty of Medicine

Director, Division Diagnostic Ultrasound
Montreal General Hospital

Acknowledgments

We give special thanks to Inge Venus, Cheryl
Meunier, and Pamela Brockway for their patience and
tireless efforts in preparing the manuscript. We are
also indebted to Doctors Richard L. Berkowitz and
Parviz Gohari for their encouragement and support,
and to Karen Moyer for her distinctly creative design.

Contents

Brief Introduction to Scanning

Although it has become customary to begin books and articles about ultrasound with a section on the basic physical principles, much of this material should now be familiar to the practitioner of ultrasound; consequently, in this chapter we wish only to deal with those aspects of the technique and physics which are not covered in the older texts and which we believe are essential to the understanding of the clinical material. In addition, we would hope to clear up misunderstanding or confusion which may have crept into the reader's mind as a result of overexposure to misinformation. Therefore, the aim of this section is not to provide an exhaustive discussion of the physical principles of ultrasound, but to deal with those problems which are currently of interest and which may be controversial. Although ultrasound is technically defined as sound of higher frequency than that which is audible to the human ear, in clinical practice it is limited to frequencies in the range from 1 to 10 million cycles/sec., that is, 1 to 10 MHz. Obstetrical ultrasound is performed in the range of 2 to 5 MHz, usually around 2 MHz. Although transmission methods of ultrasonic imaging are being developed, they are not yet of clinical value; current modes of examination employ reflected ultrasound, so-called echography. In this method, echoes returning from reflecting surfaces within the body are detected and analyzed. As the transmitted pulse from the transducer traverses the body, energy is reflected back toward the transducer from various tissue interfaces. The amount of energy which is reflected at each of these interfaces depends upon the orientation of the reflecting interface and the difference in acoustic impedance of the tissues at the interface. With current systems the same transducer is used both for transmitting and receiving. This is possible because the duration of each pulse is small compared to the time between pulses. (Systems usually employ 1000/sec. with a pulse of about 1 μsec.). There are several methods of detecting and displaying the reflected ultrasonic information. These methods will be briefly reviewed. They include A-mode, B-mode, M-mode, and B-scanning.

In A-mode, or amplitude modulation, echoes are displayed as vertical spikes along the baseline of the cathode ray tube, with the height of the spike being related to the amplitude of the detected echo. In B-mode, or brightness modulation, instead of being displayed as vertical spikes, the amplitude is represented by a spot of light on the cathode ray tube, the brightness of which is related to the intensity of the reflected echo.

B-mode is used for two-dimensional scanning or echotomography (B-scanning) and is also used for time-motion studies (M-mode). The latter application is primarily in the field of cardiology.

A-mode or amplitude modulation is a valuable clinical tool in ultrasound. The dynamic range which one can display with A-mode is greater than that which can be displayed with any form of intensity modulation. Unfortunately, the anatomical information provided by a single beam of sound is difficult to interpret and is susceptible to change produced by slight angulation of the transducer which changes the orientation of the reflecting surface to the sound beam. Therefore, the exclusive use of A-mode in ultrasonic diagnosis has practically disappeared. Modern ultrasonic diagnosis, with the exception of echoencephalography, in which a limited number of well-defined structures is being examined, and echocardiography, in which the anatomical structures being examined have characteristic motion patterns, is primarily B-scanning. It is useful to have A-mode available in conjunction with B-scanning. When the two methods are used simultaneously, the B-scan is the source of anatomical information while the A-mode representation may be used for a measurement of amplitude and distance. Thus, for example, one locates the biparietal diameter by B-scanning; but one may wish to measure the biparietal diameter using the A-mode technique.

There are a variety of ways of producing B-scans. The most commonly used in obstetrical practice is the compound contact B-scan. It is obtained by moving the transducer over the surface of the body and displaying the echoes in B-mode. However, the location and direction of the baseline must accurately follow that of the transducer. Thus the transducer arm has sine-cosine potentiometers at its joints which provide positional and directional information. (Newer instruments have been introduced which use digital rather than analog position sensors.) The operator applies a coupling medium such as mineral oil or jelly to the patient's skin and moves the transducer on the skin producing an image on a cathode ray tube.

The operator of the machine has considerable leeway in the choice of motions that he may use to examine the patient. Most commonly a group of overlapping sectors or arcs is put together to form a compound scan. This procedure has the advantage of providing a maximal amount of information about acoustic interfaces since the tissues are approached from a variety of angles. It should be remembered, however, that the more complex the motion performed by the examiner, the longer is the time required to produce a scan.

Slowness is particularly disadvantageous in obstetrics since one is dealing with a moving fetus. Another disadvantage of a complex scanning motion is that artifacts can be introduced which depend upon the number of times a particular tissue is scanned, how long the transducer is held in a particular position, and other variables of operator technique. Even with the best possible technique, compound scanning may obscure useful clues which are available from simple scans such as acoustic shadows. The fundamental difficulty with B-scanning is that one is always dealing with a slice or tomogram. With manually operated equipment it is not feasible to produce every possible slice in every possible direction so as to reconstruct a three-dimensional picture of the relevant anatomy. Such techniques are available in very specialized areas of ultrasonic diagnosis such as ophthalmology where slices can be made at 0.5-mm. intervals. It is also possible with elaborate equipment containing multiple mechanized transducers, such as the Octoson scanner of Kossoff, to produce multiple tomographic sections in a short time. For the clinician using equipment which is now commercially available, a selection of tomographic sections illustrating the anatomical and pathological features which he wishes to see must somehow be culled from the infinite number of sections which is theoretically obtainable. How does one get around this problem? The prescription which is observed in most laboratories is to insist upon cuts at specific intervals (often 0.5 cm) in both sagittal and horizontal planes from the pubis to the umbilicus or xyphoid. There are three strong arguments against this procedure:

1. The body is not laid out according to Cartesian coordinates.
2. Motion may occur during the examination.
3. It is wasteful and time-consuming.

Therefore, we suggest the use of some form of rapid or so-called "real-time" ultrasonic tomography in combination with traditional contact compound scanning in order to make an intelligent assessment of three-dimensional anatomy, observe moving structure, and properly select clinically useful anatomical cross sections. Compound scanning can then be reserved for a detailed look at certain sections after a bird's eye view has been obtained. Since there has been relatively little interest in real-time scanning in North America, a more detailed discussion of the commercially available methods of real-time B-scanning is necessary.

Real-time ultrasound

The earliest real-time scanner which became commercially available was the Siemens Vidoson. This machine was introduced in 1967, and excellent obstetrical work has been accomplished, primarily in Germany. It contains two transducers which lie at the focus of a parabolic acoustic mirror and rotate at about 7.5 times/sec. (Figure 1). The sound is reflected from the transducer to the acoustic mirror and then in a direction which is perpendicular to the scanning plane. The transducers and parabolic mirror are enclosed in a water bath so that the sound must traverse the water bath before entering the patient and re-traverse the water bath after being reflected from the patient. The use of a water bath improves the geometry of the sound beam and reduces reverberating echoes, but it limits the repetition rate. In this sytem, a linear scan is obtained about 15 times/sec.

Figure 1

The transducers rotate at the focus of a parabolic mirror. The geometry of the mirror is such that all the scan lines are parallel to each other and at right angles to the patient.

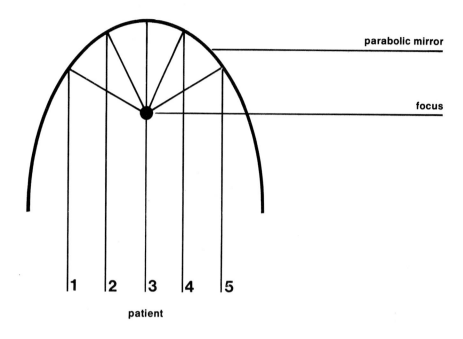

parabolic mirror

focus

1   2   3   4   5

patient

Another type of real-time scanner which is currently commercially available for use in obstetrical ultrasound is manufactured by an American company, ADR. It contains an array of 64 small transducers (Figure 2). In order to improve the geometry of the beam, the transducers are fired four at a time in a sequence which permits 40 images/sec. In both of these methods a simple linear scan is produced, and some information may be lost which could have been obtained by compound scanning because reflections which are off axis are not received. However, the need for compounding is not as great as many people assume. This is particularly true if the equipment which one uses is capable of displaying echoes of many different intensities, i.e., it has gray scale. When gray scale is available the echoes which arise from parenchymal tissue structures, the elements of which are small compared to the wave length of the sound, are not lost. These small echoes do not depend upon the angle of the beam; that is, they are not specular. For the majority of obstetrical problems, rapid simple scanning is adequate. It permits one to identify the fetus, the placenta, and the amniotic cavity. By moving the scanner in a plane which runs from the fetal head through the fetal thorax and abdomen, the position of the fetus is readily ascertained. Whether the fetus is alive or dead is easily determined by looking for fetal motion and the fetal heart beat. Since one can identify anatomical features of the fetus quickly, it is not difficult to find the proper sections from which to obtain measurements of the fetal head, the fetal thorax, the fetal abdomen, or the length of the fetus. For the experienced user, real-time scanning provides a large amount of information in a short time and permits a dynamic assessment of three-dimensional anatomy.

Figure 2

Diagram indicating the pattern of transducer firing in ADR real-time instrument. Sequence starts at left and each transducer fires 40 times/sec. Transducers are fired in groups of four.

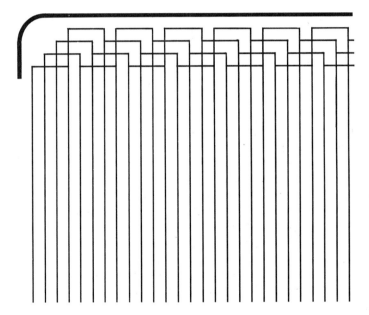

As various clinical problems are discussed in this text, the complementary use of real-time scanning and compound contact scanning will be presented as well as the advantages and disadvantages of each. In this introductory section it is, however, worthwhile to mention just a few examples illustrating the necessity of real-time scanning. The problem of fetal life has already been mentioned, and with a real-time scanner fetal motion may be observed as early as 8 weeks. The identification of the placenta and the determination of whether it crosses the cervix do not, at first glance, appear to be problems which require real-time scanning for a solution. However, it occasionally happens that a fetal limb is positioned in such a way that it is difficult to distinguish from placenta. By observing its motion this distinction can be made. When one sees a fetal limb moving about in amniotic fluid adjacent to the cervix, it is clear that no placenta could occupy that space, and the diagnosis of a marginal placenta previa can be discarded with confidence. Fetal respiration has been described using A-mode methods. However, A-mode methods are obviously cumbersome and susceptible to misinterpretation and artifacts. Real-time imaging is a preferable method of observing fetal respiration. Anyone who has spent a great deal of time attempting to interpret the images obtained on a compound scanner in a case of twins or triplets will readily appreciate the enormous convenience of getting an overview of the whole uterus, counting the number of heads and bodies, and piecing them together into a coherent three-dimensional image.

Gray scale

Another technical concept which needs to be clarified is that of gray scale. In performing a B-scan, one assumes that the relative reflectivity of the different acoustical interfaces has been appropriately represented on the cathode ray tube by points of light, the brightness of each of which corresponds to the intensity of the echo from the anatomical surface. (Even in A-mode work, this correspondence may be distorted. Many commercially available systems do not have adequate logarithmic compression of echoes and may saturate the amplifier, making all strong echoes appear to be equal.) If one takes a conventional compound contact scanner and moves the transducer rapidly over the patient with the cathode ray tube set in a non-storage mode, some intensity modulation can be obtained. However, when a storage tube is used, an arbitrary cut-off level is made below which no echoes are represented and above which all echoes are of the same brightness. The storage tube is capable of representing only two levels, on and off. Thus, it is called "bistable" (Figure 3).

Before 1974 no scanner was available on the North American market in which compound contact scanning could be performed with any gray scale. Some methods had been developed which utilized non-storage oscilloscopes and long exposure photographic techniques. However, these were extremely cumbersome and required the technique of a violin virtuoso. Beginning in 1974, an important technological development was introduced to the ultrasound market. This development was the scan converter. The scan converter is a device containing a matrix of elements, generally 1000 × 1000, each of which is capable of exhibiting several levels of intensity. By coupling the scan converter to the cathode ray tube, it became possible to use compound contact scanning in a storage mode and to obtain images with a wide dynamic range of intensity modulation.

Figure 3

Amplitude of reflected echoes are represented by the height of each spike. Those echoes of amplitude above preset threshold are stored. Those echoes which are below threshold are rejected. The displayed echoes are the same brightness, regardless of the amplitude of the reflected sound.

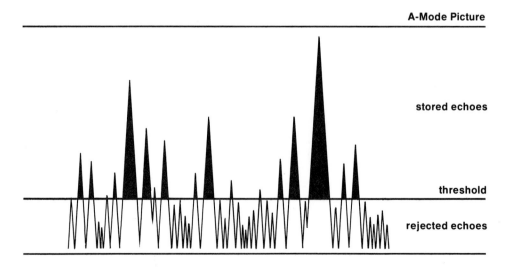

A-Mode Picture

stored echoes

threshold

rejected echoes

It should be pointed out that the real-time instruments do not require a scan converter since they do not use a storage tube. Even the early real-time instruments possessed some gray scale. Another feature of the scan converter which is useful is that an individual element, having received a certain signal, will not respond to a subsequent signal unless it is stronger than that of the first. This feature prevents summation of weak echoes producing the appearance of strong echoes. However, it is subject to abuse and does not prevent an unduly long scan from degrading resolution when motion has occurred.

The method by which echoes of different intensity are displayed as different levels of gray in the scan converter varies with each manufacturer. (Many refinements of scanner converter technique are in development by various manufacturers.) Before scan converters were introduced, the bleeding of the image on the storage oscilloscope was so severe that most manufacturers used what was known as ''leading edge'' presentation. That is, when a pulse returning from a particular structure is a millimeter or more in width, only the first fraction of a millimeter was displayed on the scope. This provided lines of minimal width which appeared to be sharply outlined. It accentuated the fundamental problem in bistable scanning of an inability to represent weak echoes, so that the anatomical quality was further degraded in such organs as the placenta and liver because almost no parenchymal texture was available. Unfortunately, some concepts that were promulgated about ultrasonic diagnosis evolved when this technique was widely used. We hope that leading edge bistable scanning has seen its day since better methods are now available to supplant it.

Leading edge detection is still used for measuring the biparietal diameter by many users of compound contact scanners. This is because the lines are fine, and the image appears to be more accurately measurable. (This problem is discussed in more detail under the section on biparietal measurement.)

The echoes returning from a structure far away from the transducer are less intense than those returning from an interface which is near the transducer because some of the sound is absorbed in the intervening tissue. Therefore, all ultrasonic instruments have a method of compensating for this physical problem. It is called time-gain compensation or TGC. (A newer method of time-gain compensation is just beginning to appear on the market in which there is selective depth compensation over 2-cm. intervals.) They also have various devices for increasing the amplification of the signals returned to the transducer, attenuating them, suppressing weak echoes below a certain threshold, and changing the energy with which the transducer is struck. Unfortunately, manufacturers are imprecise about the function of each of the dials on ultrasound machines. It also seems that the literature is full of contradictory statements as to the proper settings of these dials for the recognition of various anatomical regions and pathological states. For the moment, the ultrasonographer is in the uncomfortable position of being required to know what the image he expects to see will look like before he can make an appropriate setting of his amplification and attenuation controls. He is somewhat helped with these problems by gray scale imaging which has simplified the manipulation of gain controls by obviating any tendency of saturating the oscilloscope and producing meaningless hash. The need for dial fiddling is reduced in real-time scanning since the visual feedback from the image is instantaneous. The operator of a contact scanner has to repeat the movement of the transducer and build up a new stored image with a new set of amplification settings, whereas the operator of a real-time scanner continues to look at a live image while he manipulates the controls.

Nonetheless, ultrasonography is not yet like radiography. A patient who is having a frontal and lateral film of the chest merely needs to stand in front of a cassette, and the technician can push a button with a high probability that a satisfactory image will be obtained. This image can be reviewed by a knowledgeable physician after it has been taken, and only rarely is the technical quality of the images unsatisfactory for interpretation.

In ultrasonography, there is a dynamic relation between the image that the ultrasonographer expects to see and the subsequent manipulation of the transducer or the machine controls that he will undertake. Therefore, he needs to have a broad knowledge of anatomy and pathology. Technicians can be trained to competently perform ultrasonic examinations, but it does not suffice to take a 2-day course offered by the manufacturer of ultrasound equipment. Fortunately, standards for certification of technicians and physicians in the field of diagnostic ultrasound are now being discussed. Also, newer equipment, particularly real-time and gray scale equipment, has removed a great deal of the hocus-pocus which used to be associated with the performance of ultrasonic examinations. We look forward to the development of equipment which will be comparable to that of the chest radiograph machine. These improvements in equipment will include automated systems for producing compound images employing mechanical scanners.

One of the refinements of technique which can be obtained with current equipment is to change the frequency of the transducers. Higher frequency transducers provide better resolution so that structures such as the fetal head are represented by finer lines. Higher frequency transducers are less subject to problems with near field reverberations. Thus, it is usually not necessary to use drastic near field attenuation, and gain controls are simplified.

The disadvantage of higher frequency transducers is that the sound is more strongly attenuated. Despite reduced penetration, many pregnant uteri can be effectively examined at 3.5 MHz rather than the conventional 2.25 MHz, and a superior image quality can be attained. The greater attenuation of high frequency sound can also be used to advantage in distinguishing cystic from solid masses, since the attenuation of the higher frequency sound by fluid remains negligible whereas it is absorbed by solid tissue (Figure 4).

Figure 4

Demonstration of white on black pictures of same fibroid using transducers of different frequency. In *A*, a 2.25 MHz transducer was used, and in *B*, where lower border of the fibroid is lost, a 3.5 MHz transducer was used.

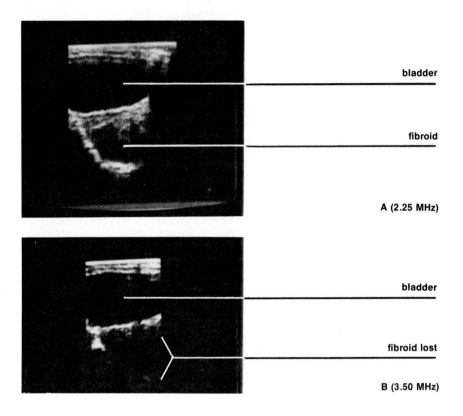

bladder

fibroid

A (2.25 MHz)

bladder

fibroid lost

B (3.50 MHz)

Measurements

Before concluding this brief section on physics and instrumentation, a few words need to be said about measurement. Some of the literature in ultrasound gives one the impression of a contest as to who can measure more accurately. We do not wish to minimize the importance of accuracy of measurement. Surely all measurements should be made as accurately as possible. However, one must be aware of the limitations imposed by the equipment and the fundamental physical principles. All measurements made with clinically available instruments depend upon the assumption that the velocity of sound in tissue is constant. This is because the measuring instrument, i.e., the cathode ray tube, has a sweep speed which is related to the velocity of sound in tissue. The amount of time required for a signal to return to the transducer is thus interpreted by the instrument as a distance. Instruments which are used in North America take as their standard a velocity of 1540 meters/sec. This velocity is not correct for certain tissues, in particular the fetal skull. However, it does not help to make an arbitrary change in velocity calibration since the exact change one should make is not precisely known, and the thickness and degree of calcification of the fetal skull do not remain constant throughout pregnancy. The accuracy of measurement also depends upon the depth resolution and lateral resolution of the instrument. The depth resolution can be no better than the wave length of the sound being employed; since a transducer of 2.5 MHz has a wave length of 0.6 mm., it does not seem reasonable to claim accuracy which is superior to that. Lateral resolution is determined by the diameter of the sonic beam at the point where the measurement is being made. The beam width, in turn, is determined by the design of the transducer and the type of focusing which is used. In all cases lateral resolution is poorer than depth resolution; but when two structures adjacent to each other laterally are not resolved, depth resolution is affected. The wave form which is produced by the transducer also affects depth resolution, and this may depend upon the energy with which the transducer is struck and the physical characteristics of the transducer backing. Finally, the resolution of the cathode ray tube, the film which is used to photograph it, and the electronic or mechanical calipers which are used to make the measurement will all affect the accuracy of the measurements. A realistic attitude toward the inherent limitations of measurement should be maintained by the ultrasonographer. No measurement is better than the ruler with which it is made.

References

1 **Goldberg, B., Kotler, M., Ziskin, M., and Waxham, R.** *Diagnostic Uses of Ultrasound.* Grune & Stratton, Inc., New York, 1975.
2 **Wells, P.N.T.** *Physical Principles of Ultrasonic Diagnosis.* Academic Press, New York, 1969.

Early Pregnancy

The best starting point for the discussion of early pregnancy is an examination of the non-pregnant uterus. It is generally recognized that an adequate ultrasonic examination of the uterus requires that the patient have a full bladder. Nonetheless, when a patient arrives without a full bladder, one is always tempted to conduct the examination in order to save time and spare the patient further inconvenience. This temptation should be resisted. The bladder must be sufficiently full so that it covers the fundus of the uterus. If the uterus tends to be anteverted, a full bladder will depress it and make its examination easier. If the uterus is retroverted, a full bladder will at least push bowel away from the fundus. Examining the patient who has an empty bladder will only lead to frustration and diagnostic errors (Figures 1a and 1b).

Figure 1a

Scanning small uterus with insufficiently full bladder.

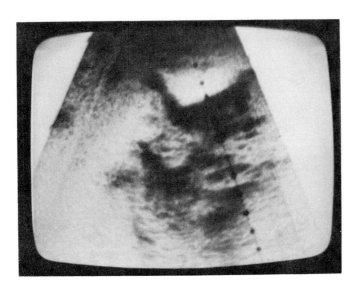

Figure 1b

Scanning with full bladder.

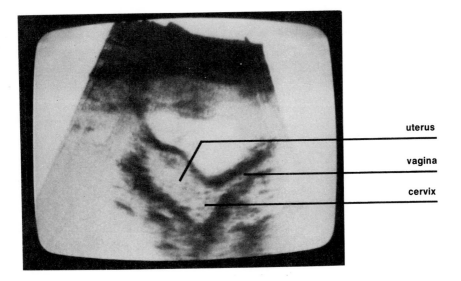

uterus

vagina

cervix

Figure 1c

Schematic representation of transverse scans at different levels of lower abdomen.

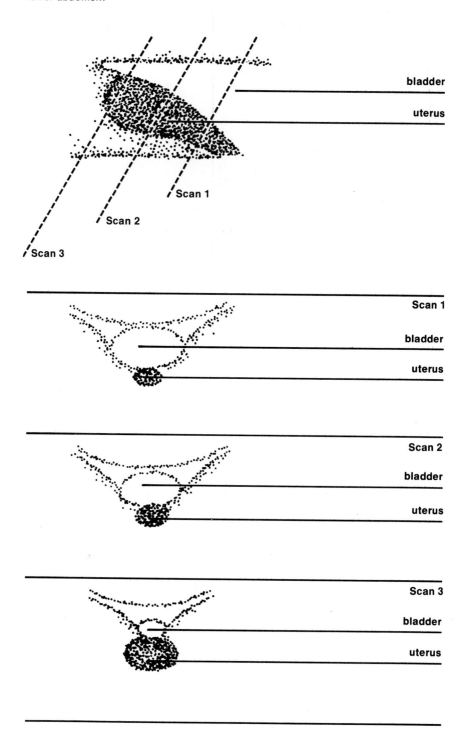

Figure 2

Linear echo in non-pregnant uterus.

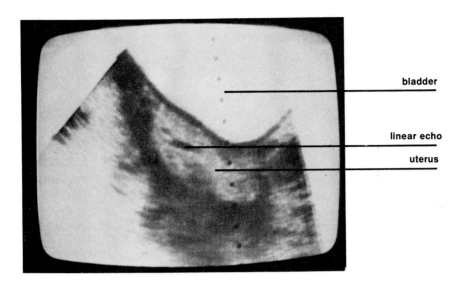

bladder

linear echo

uterus

The widest portion of the bladder lies above the narrowest portion of the uterus, the cervix. As one moves superiorly, the bladder becomes narrower as the uterus becomes wider (Figure 1c). With equipment which has wide dynamic range (gray scale), the uterine cervix and fundus can be clearly identified. Occasionally, a centrally located linear echo is observed in the uterus either at the level of the cervix or in the fundus. Presumably, this represents the interface between adjacent levels of endometrium (Figure 2). It should not be mistaken for an intrauterine device. (Intrauterine devices of various types are identified by their relatively strong interfaces and unbiological geometry.)

Figure 3
Very early gestation.

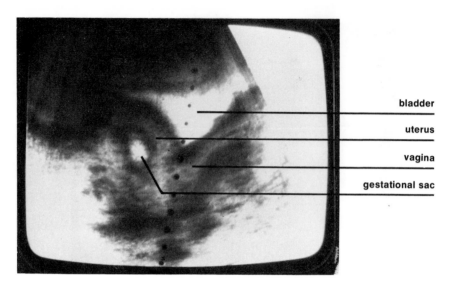

bladder

uterus

vagina

gestational sac

The diagnosis of pregnancy can be made about 5 to 6 weeks after the last menstrual period. A rounded fluid-containing sac is seen in the uterus which has been called the gestational sac (Figure 3). Embryologically, it consists of a combination of the chorionic and aminotic cavities (primarily the former) and is surrounded by chorionic villi and decidual reaction. These surrounding structures were not appreciated in the early literature because leading edge bistable equipment was used, and therefore only the periphery of the fluid-containing cavity was seen. Consequently, it was concluded that one could identify the site of implantation by identifying that wall of the uterus lying adjacent to the gestational sac.

In fact, the thicker parts of the chorion are likely to be farther from the wall of the uterus because the decidual reaction at the site of implantation is more intense. Therefore, conclusions about the site of implantation based on proximity to a uterine wall are incorrect. The chorion soon divides into two portions, the chorion frondosum and the chorion laeve (Figure 4). The chorion frondosum forms the primordial placenta, which is separated from the uterine wall by decidua basalis.

Figure 4

Illustration of components of early pregnancy A.
As pregnancy progresses placenta occupies a fundal position B.

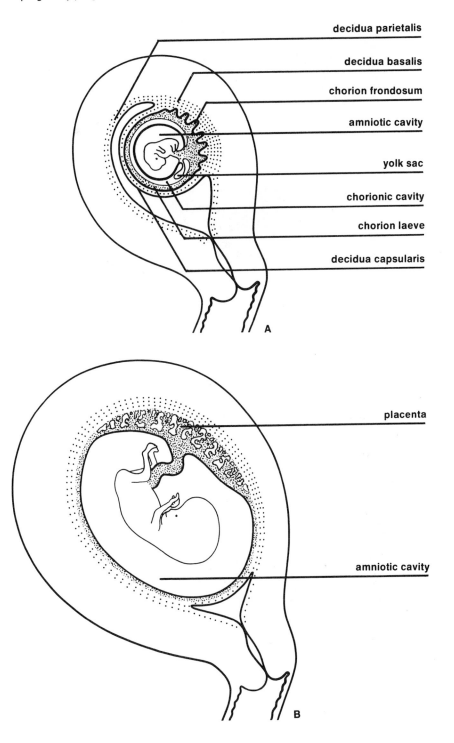

decidua parietalis

decidua basalis

chorion frondosum

amniotic cavity

yolk sac

chorionic cavity

chorion laeve

decidua capsularis

A

placenta

amniotic cavity

B

Figure 5

Seven-week gestation.

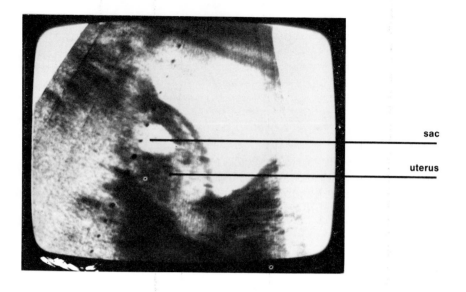

sac

uterus

Figure 6

Eight-week pregnancy with embryo.

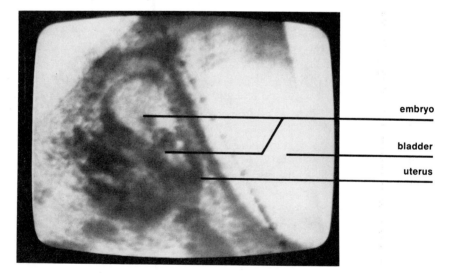

embryo

bladder

uterus

At about 8 weeks after the last menstrual period, the disk-like shape of the gestation can be appreciated. The gestational sac usually has a thin wall facing the uterine cavity and a thick wall attached to the uterus (Figure 5). At 8 weeks, one should be able to see an embryo in the amniotic cavity, and with real-time equipment motion may be perceived (Figure 6). The gestational sac continues to grow and usually fills the entire uterine cavity at about the 11th week. The placenta can frequently be identified as early as the eighth week but is relatively easy to see by the 11th or 12th week. By the 10th week, embryonic activity is consistently noted, and it is even possible to identify the fetal heart beat using high speed real-time equipment. Beyond 12 weeks, no difficulty should be encountered in measuring the fetal head or identifying the fetal heart.

Threatened or missed abortion

Twenty percent of pregnant women bleed vaginally in the first trimester, but less than half of these are destined to abort. If abortion is preceded by sudden and profuse bleeding, often it must be dealt with under poorly controlled conditions. In order to avoid this potentially hazardous emergency situation, some investigators have attempted to use ultrasound to predict which jeopardized pregnancy will abort. Low-lying, ill-defined, and double gestational sacs have been reported to correlate with an unfavorable outcome. Others have associated ill-defined placentas and small-for-dates uteri and gestational sacs with abortion. In our experience none of these criteria consistently correlates with the outcome of pregnancy. The absence of an embryo in the gestational sac after about 8 weeks is a reliable finding. Before one can conclude that the gestational sac contains no embryo, however, it must be thoroughly scanned. Rapid non-storage scanning or real-time scanning is helpful in insuring that no portion of the chorionic cavity has been overlooked. Even when an embryo is present, it cannot be concluded that the gestation is viable unless the embryo is observed to move.

Figure 7

Transverse scan of missed abortion.
In this case there was no growth of the uterus.
Note flattened gestational sac.

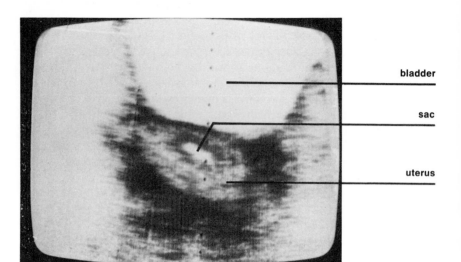

bladder

sac

uterus

Doubt about the viability of a gestation can be resolved if the fetal heart can be detected. There are three methods of detecting the fetal heart. The easiest method is to use real-time equipment. The Siemens Vidoson produces 15 images/sec., and the heart can be reliably seen at 12 weeks. With the ADR multitransducer device there are 40 images/sec., and we have observed and cinegraphically recorded the heart as early as 10 weeks. Doppler ultrasound detects the heart as early as 8 weeks and, in experienced hands, is reliable at 12 weeks. M-mode echocardiography has been reported by Robinson to be reliable as early as 6 weeks; but it is a tedious procedure, too tedious for general use in the first trimester. We have been unable to consistently obtain M-mode tracings of the fetal heart in the first trimester, but this is probably due to the fact that our equipment is different from that used by Robinson. *In difficult cases a repeat scan should be carried out in about 1 week; if no change has occurred or the gestation has regressed, lingering uncertainty will be dispelled* (Figure 7).

When abortion has already occurred, multiple disorganized echoes are seen within the uterus. If abortion has been complete, the uterus may be indistinguishable from a non-pregnant uterus except for its size. The difference between incomplete abortion and missed abortion is perhaps more theological than practical, but in a missed abortion one is likely to see a gestation which is not in correspondence with the patient's dates and which shows no signs of life.

Ectopic pregnancy

One of the serious problems with which one is commonly faced in obstetrical and gynecological ultrasonography is the suspected diagnosis of an ectopic pregnancy. Patients with a variety of clinical problems are sent for ultrasonic diagnosis to exclude an ectopic pregnancy. These include dysmenorrhea, pelvic inflammatory disease, ovarian cyst complicating pregnancy, twisted ovarian cyst, and incomplete abortion. The accuracy with which the diagnosis of ectopic pregnancy can be made by ultrasound is controversial. The most common condition confused with ectopic pregnancy is an intrauterine pregnancy with a corpus luteum cyst of the ovary (Figure 8). In both conditions the patient presents with lower abdominal pain, positive pregnancy test, and a tender adnexal mass. Blood may even be aspirated from the cul-de-sac. If an intrauterine gestation can be demonstrated, the diagnosis of ectopic pregnancy can almost certainly be excluded since it is extremely rare to encounter a twin pregnancy in a fallopian tube. If the uterus is small or slightly enlarged, an intrauterine gestation cannot be completely ruled out since the patient's dates may be in error, and a very early pregnancy may be present. If the patient has a tender abdomen, a positive pregnancy test, an enlarged uterus, and a gestational sac is not seen, a laparoscopy should be performed. The diagnosis of an ectopic pregnancy cannot be excluded simply because an extrauterine gestation has not been identified. In about one-third of ectopic pregnancies the urine pregnancy test is negative. However, analysis of serum beta subunit of chorionic gonadotropin is always positive. Ectopic or intrauterine gonadotropin activity can persist for weeks after abortion.

Figure 8
Early pregnancy with corpus luteum cyst.

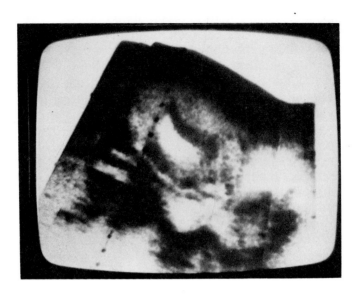

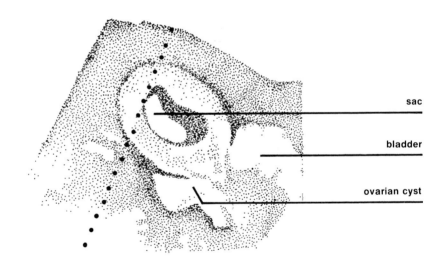

Figure 9a

Transverse scan of ectopic gestation.

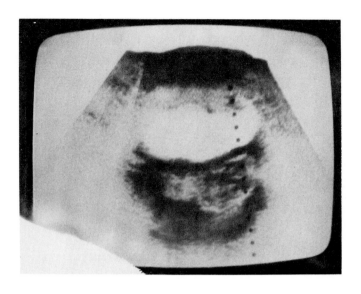

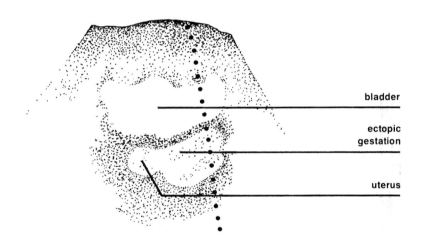

bladder

ectopic
gestation

uterus

Figure 9b
Ectopic pregnancy with gestation sac in fallopian tube.

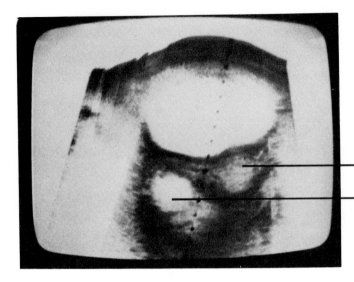

uterus

gestation sac

In some ectopic gestations, an abnormal, relatively solid mass is identified adjacent to the uterus (Figure 9a). It may lie superior to the uterus, lateral to it, or inferiorly in the cul-de-sac (Figure 9b). The mass may have the configuration of an early gestational sac; or, in the case of a chronic ectopic abortion, it may simply be a collection of blood (pelvic hematocele). Displacement of the uterus or blood in the cul-de-sac (Figure 10) may be present when no well-defined mass is identified. Corpus luteum cysts also accompany ectopic gestations.

One pitfall which should be avoided is the misidentification of a loop of bowel lying above the uterine fundus as an ectopic gestation, an error which is more likely to be made if the bladder is not full enough to displace bowel away from the fundus. When real-time equipment is available such loops of bowel can be identified by gas transport within them producing characteristic motion echoes. The gas passes through fluid-filled loops of bowel and is readily observed due to its high acoustic reflectivity.

Figure 10

Blood in cul-de-sac in ectopic gestation.

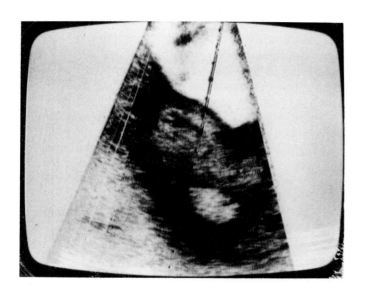

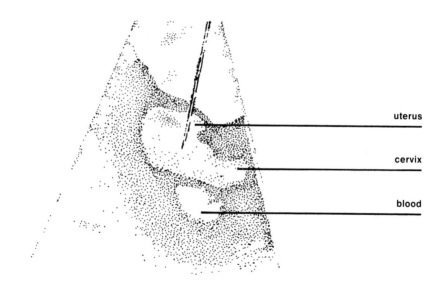

uterus

cervix

blood

Hydatidiform mole

Hydatidiform mole is an important complication of early pregnancy, and ultrasound has become the definitive means of diagnosis. In roughly 50% of cases the uterus is larger than would be anticipated from menstrual history. The ultrasonic appearance of a mole reflects the gross pathological appearance. That is, the individual solid elements are separated by fluid spaces. Thus, a mole does not look like a normal placenta, but resembles an edematous placenta (Figure 11). Although the typical mole is easy to identify, about one-third of moles have an atypical appearance because they contain large blood clots or areas of cystic degeneration (Figure 12). Thus, they resemble incomplete abortions. With currently available ultrasonic equipment, there is no reliable way of distinguishing an atypical mole from an incomplete abortion. The history, physical findings, and chorionic gonadotropin levels must be considered before one diagnoses a hydatidiform mole. Theca lutein cysts may develop in response to the persistently high titers of chorionic gonadotropin, and this finding may aid the ultrasonographer in the diagnosis of a mole. It has been reported, even in the recent literature, that a mistaken diagnosis of a mole can be made by a cut through the placenta. This error should be avoided if proper scanning technique is employed. One must make a large number of slices in order to examine the entire uterus. This can be expeditiously accomplished by the use of rapid scanning methods, preferably real-time.

When the patient with a mole is sent for ultrasonic examination, the diagnosis is often not suspected. It is obviously in the best interest of the patient that the diagnosis of mole be made as early as possible. Therefore, the patient should be sent for ultrasonic examination early if suggestive symptoms are present.

The most common symptoms associated with a mole are vaginal bleeding with or without cramping in a patient presumed to be pregnant and excessive vomiting in early pregnancy. The most common finding on pelvic examination is a firm uterus that is disporportionately large for dates (although an occasional patient will have a mole contained within a small uterus). Once the diagnosis is made by ultrasound, it is imperative that the ultrasonographer's report be explicit and leave no room for procrastination. It is not acceptable to suspect a diagnosis of a mole and request another ultrasound after an interval of time. An unwary clinician may be comforted by the subsequent uterine enlargement and positive pregnancy test.

Figure 11
Typical hydatidiform mole.

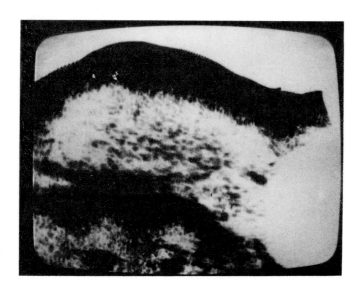

Figure 12
Atypical mole.

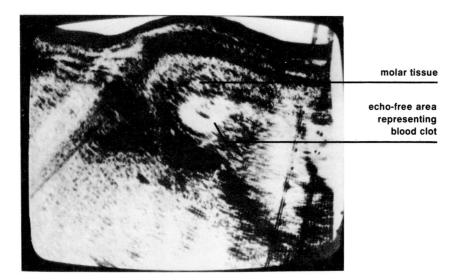

molar tissue

echo-free area
representing
blood clot

Figure 13
Incomplete abortion resembling mole.

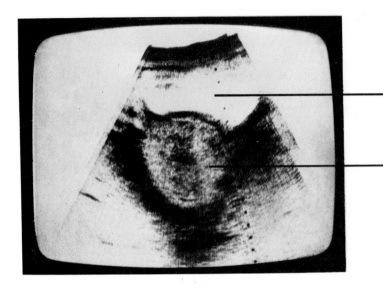

bladder

uterus

In addition to the problem of mole masquerading as incomplete abortion, one is occasionally confronted with an incomplete abortion resembling a mole (Figure 13). Rarely, a uterine leiomyoma may also mimic a mole. There is no way to distinguish a choriocarcinoma from a mole with ultrasound.

Adnexal masses

A common problem in the first trimester is the association of ovarian and uterine masses. Ovarian cysts are frequently seen in the first trimester, and the patient is often referred with a suspected diagnosis of ectopic gestation (see Figure 8). The ultrasonographer can play an important role in this situation by demonstrating a normal intrauterine gestation associated with an ovarian cyst, thus excluding the diagnosis of an ectopic gestation. The · evolution of the cyst may be followed throughout the pregnancy. Uterine fibroids are also seen together with early pregnancies. Under these circumstances they are relatively echo-free and tend to displace the gestation (Figure 14). It is particularly characteristic to see the placenta displaced from the uterine wall by a fibroid.

Uterine fibroids may increase enormously in size under hormonal stimulation. As the pregnancy progresses, the fibroid may outgrow its blood supply resulting in cystic necrosis of the center of the

Figure 14
Supracervical fibroid and early gestation.

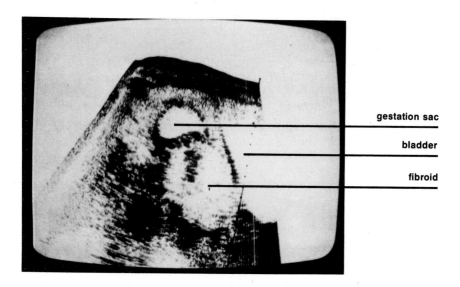

gestation sac

bladder

fibroid

myoma. Although fibroids resemble cysts ultrasonically, the characteristic differences between cysts and solid tumors remain applicable. That is, the attenuation of sound by a fibroid is greater than that which occurs in cysts, and the walls are not as clearly defined. Use of higher frequency transducers is helpful in making this distinction.

A cystic teratoma or dermoid cyst is another tumor associated with pregnancy. Its features are variable because of the wide variety of gross pathological appearance of this tumor (see Chapter 8 on "Gynecology").

Pregnancy with intrauterine devices

An IUD is easily located by ultrasound in a non-pregnant uterus. Occasionally, a patient with an intrauterine device becomes pregnant, and the ultrasonographer is called upon to locate the IUD. In our experience in these cases it is extremely difficult to identify the IUD after the first trimester. Often the device attaches itself to the placenta or uterine wall. As the uterus grows, the IUD is drawn into the cavity and attains a lateral position between uterine wall and membranes. In this position it is ultrasonically lost. Therefore, the inability to identify an intrauterine device in a pregnant patient does not cause the same concern that it does in a non-pregnant patient. In the latter, the possibility that it has perforated the uterine cavity must be considered. An additional problem is posed by the fact that intrauterine contraceptive devices are sometimes associated with ectopic gestations and pelvic inflammatory disease. Also the size and configuration of IUD's change as medical science progresses. The steel ring has given way to the loop and spiral. The newest product, the copper-7 IUD, is quite difficult to locate because of its size and shape. Some authors have recommended that ultrasound not be used in patients with copper IUD's since heat may be produced from the interaction of mechanical energy and the copper.

References

1 **Blackwell, R.J., Shirley, I., Earman, D. J., and Michael, C. A.** Ultrasonic "B" scanning as a pregnancy test after less than six weeks amenorrhoea. Br. J. Obstet. Gynaecol. 82:108, 1975.

2 **Donald, I., Morley, P., and Barnett, E.** The diagnosis of blighted ovum by sonar. J. Obstet. Gynaecol. Br. Commonw. 79:304, 1972.

3 **Drumm, J. E., and Clinch, J.** Ultrasound in management of clinically diagnosed threatened abortion. Br. Med. J. 02(5968):424, 1975.

4 **Hellman, L. M., Kobayashi, M., and Cromb, E.** Ultrasonic diagnosis of embryonic malformations. Am. J. Obstet. Gynecol. 115:615, 1973.

5 **Jouppila, P.** Ultrasound in the diagnosis of early pregnancy and its complications. Acta Obstet. Gynecol. Scand. (Suppl.) 15:3, 1971.

6 **Kohorn, E., and Kaufman, M.** Sonar in the first trimester of pregnancy. Obstet. Gynecol. 44:473, 1974.

7 **Leopold, G. R.** Diagnostic ultrasound in the detection of molar pregnancy. Radiology 98:171, 1971.

8 **Robinson, H. P.** Gestation sac: volumes as determined by sonar in the first trimester of pregnancy. Br. J. Obstet. Gynaecol. 82:100, 1975.

9 **Robinson, H. P.** Sonar measurement of fetal crown-rump length as means of assessing maturity in first trimester of pregnancy. Br. Med. J. 4:28, 1973.

10 **Sauvage, J. P., Crane, J. P., and Kopta, M. M.** Difficulties in the ultrasonic diagnosis of hydatidiform mole. Obstet. Gynecol. 44:546, 1974.

11 **Weill, F., Heitz, P., Fega, R., and Becker, J. C.** Problems in the ultrasonic diagnosis of hydatidiform mole. J. Radiol. Electrol. Med. Nucl. 53:697, 1972.

12 **Weiss, P. A., and Lichtenegger, W.** Differential diagnostic difficulties in the ultrasonographic diagnosis of hydatidiform mole (author's transl). Geburtshilfe Frauenheilkd. 34:633, 1974.

Estimation of Gestational Age

3

As might be surmised from the previous chapter on the early gestation, gestational age between 6 and 12 weeks can be estimated from the size of the gestational sac. Robinson has made measurements of the volume of the gestational sac; although these represent an improvement, it would appear that such measurements are beyond the constraints of time imposed in the average laboratory. Measurements of the uterus have also been made, but the variability of shape of the uterus in early pregnancy makes the selection of standard measurements difficult. Another method which has been used to estimate gestational age is crown-rump length. Robinson has shown that the length varies from 10 mm. at 7 weeks to 85 mm. at 14 weeks (see Appendix). Because of the infinite variety of positions in which the very mobile fetus may lie in early gestations, the measurement of crown-rump length is difficult to make using contact equipment. Robinson employed multiple sections from which he selected the proper obliquity for measurement of the crown-rump length. His data show a fetal length-maturity curve which is quite impressive with an accuracy of plus or minus 3 days. Crown-rump length can be measured with less difficulty when high resolution real-time equipment is used to locate the proper scanning plane (Figures 1 and 2).

Although crown-rump length is undoubtedly the most accurate way of dating gestations up to 12 weeks, the problem of dating should be kept in clinical perspective. The period of time from the formation of the gestational sac until the fetal head is measured is 6 weeks. It is easy to divide this into 2-week periods by observing the fraction of the uterus which is filled by the gestation. If the six-week gestation is taken to be a sac of about 2 cm. in size, the 8-week gestation to be a larger sac filling approximately two-thirds of the uterine cavity, and the 10-week gestation to be a sac filling the entire uterine cavity with a diameter of

Figure 1

Fetal length at 9 weeks.
Transverse scan in gray scale.

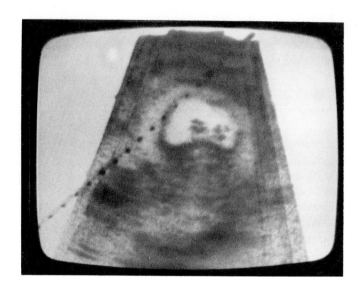

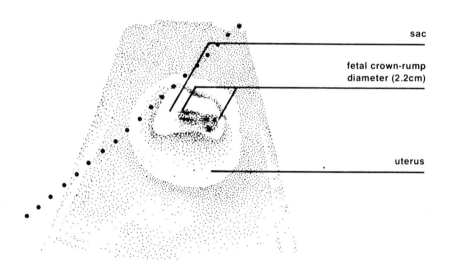

sac

fetal crown-rump
diameter (2.2cm)

uterus

Figure 2
Fetal length at 11 weeks.
Longitudinal scan in gray scale.

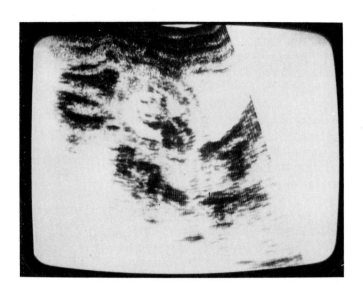

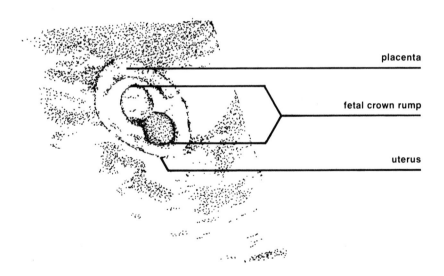

approximately 5 cm., the problem is simplified. It must be remembered, however, that there is variability between patients in proportion of sac size to uterine size, and this is not the best way to estimate gestation. Using modern equipment, no difficulty should be encountered in measuring the fetal head at 12 weeks (Figure 3), and the fetal biparietal diameter is an excellent means of estimating fetal age in the second trimester. In our opinion, this strategy of dating is generally acceptable in the first trimester since the uncertainty of dating is usually a multiple of 4 weeks. The identification and measurement of the fetal head at the 12th week requires equipment with high resolution and dynamic range. Since fetal movement is very active, real-time equipment is helpful.

The biparietal diameter of the fetal skull is an excellent means of estimation of gestational age in the second trimester because the measurement is subject to relatively little error, and there is a close correlation between biparietal diameter and gestational age. The fetal skull is growing rapidly and is relatively thin. Thus, in the early second trimester a measurement error of 5 mm. may correspond to only 1 week of growth, and the thinness of the fetal skull makes correction for velocity of sound in bone unnecessary. Another advantage of a thin fetal skull is that there is no ambiguity about the points from which measurements should be made. As the gestation progresses, the rate of fetal growth is reduced while the accuracy of measurement is not improved. In addition, the correlation of biparietal diameter to maturity is reduced as the pregnancy advances. Thus, the more advanced the pregnancy, the less reliable is the dating by biparietal diameter. In a patient in whom there is risk of growth retardation, measurement of the fetal head should begin in the second trimester. Since the standard error of measurement of the biparietal diameter is about 2 mm., and the growth of the biparietal diameter falls to about 1.5 mm./week in the last trimester, serial measurements of the biparietal diameter in the third trimester do not provide an adequate method of monitoring growth retardation. Moreover, as will be discussed later in a subsequent chapter on fetal growth and development, the fetal head may continue to grow normally when there is placental insufficiency whereas the body undergoes growth retardation. Retardation of fetal head growth occurs relatively late in the course of placental insufficiency.

Figure 3

Biparietal diameter at 12 weeks.
Sagittal scan.

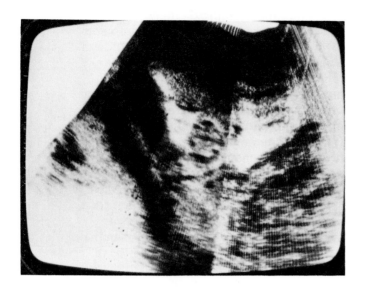

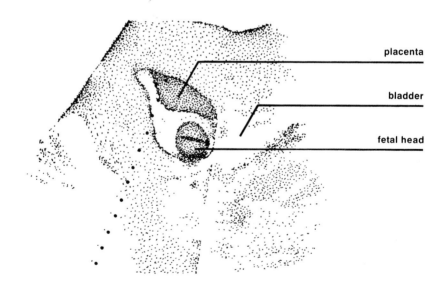

placenta

bladder

fetal head

If we accept as the standard error between measurements of the skull approximately 2 mm., in order to say with 95% confidence that the change is not due to a measuring error, this change must be at least 1.68 × 2 mm., that is, approximately 3.4 mm. Assuming that we have made two fetal measurements separated by a certain interval of time and no growth of the fetal head has been observed, it is necessary that the predicted difference between the two measurements be greater than 3.4 mm. before we can conclude that there has been growth retardation. In the fourth month of pregnancy the rate of growth is 5 mm./week. Thus, if one were to measure no growth between measurements made a week apart, this result would have less than 5% probability of being due to a measuring error. In the fifth month the rate of growth is 3.6 mm./week, so that zero growth between two weekly measurements would have statistical significance. If, however, only 0.3 mm. of growth had occurred, one would have to wait a longer period of time before concluding that there was a high probability of growth retardation. In the eighth month, when the rate of growth is 2.3 mm./week, zero growth in 2 weeks could be considered significant; but only 1.2 mm. of growth in 2 weeks would still be borderline.

In the 10th month, when growth is only 1.4 mm./week or less, even 2 weeks without apparent growth cannot be considered significant. (The reader is referred to the excellent article by Davison et al. for a complete and rigorous discussion of the statistical problem involved in assessing fetal age and growth by means of the biparietal diameter.)

The above simplified examples indicate the importance of dating a pregnancy as early as possible and following it from the fourth month in patients with risk of growth retardation. If one could be confident that a measurement of less than 2 mm. were the standard difference error, then the diagnosis of failure of growth of the fetal head could be made in a correspondingly shorter time. However, 2 mm. is probably what can be expected in the average careful laboratory even when A-mode measurements are used.

A method which the individual user can employ to test his own reliability has been proposed by Davison. That is, a series of measurements is made on the same patient 24 hours apart. They must, of course, be made without knowledge of the previous measurement. Since it can be assumed that no growth has occurred during the 24-hour period, the standard deviation of the difference between the two measurements can be used as the "between occasion error."

It has become a common practice in most hospitals to document fetal maturity before elective induction or cesarean section is carried out. Although the accuracy of ultrasonic dating is best in early gestations, the ultrasonographer is most frequently confronted with the task of determining fetal maturity a few days before interruption of pregnancy is contemplated. There certainly is some correlation between biparietal diameter and fetal maturity in late gestation so that the use of biparietal diameter measurements alone has diminished the incidence of premature deliveries. In our experience, however, the biparietal diameter is a misleading index of maturity in very large babies or infants of diabetic mothers. Therefore, if possible, we prefer to perform an amniocentesis to document pulmonic maturity before elective interruption of pregnancy and date the pregnancy by the 24th week with a biparietal measurement. If the biparietal diameter (BPD) is less than 8.7 cm. (our mean BPD for 37 weeks) and there is no evidence of intrauterine growth retardation, the amniocentesis is postponed for 1 week. Previously, if the ultrasound scan suggested that an amniocentesis would be hazardous and there was no evidence of maternal diabetes, we felt it was generally safe to interrupt the pregnancy when the biparietal diameter was 9 cm. or above. In a recent study, however, we were surprised to find that 29% of fetuses with BPD's of 9 or more had immature lecithin-sphingomyelin (L/S) ratios (less than 2). When the BPD was 8.7 to 9 cm., 40% of these babies had immature L/S ratios. These biparietal diameters are all based on leading edge measurements. For those using full thickness of distal scalp and those using 1600 m./sec. sound velocity, measurements will be about 3 mm. larger. Since these babies were not delivered at that point, it was impossible to determine whether any of them would have developed respiratory distress syndrome (RDS). Despite the rather high incidence of immature L/S ratios with BPD's of greater than 9, one author suspects that a BPD compatible with 38 weeks still correlates well with fetal lung maturity since he has not seen such a baby develop RDS. On the other hand (and this will be discussed in Chapter 7), L/S ratios of less than 2 are often noted prior to the birth of a pulmonically mature infant.

The literature is replete with reports of accuracy of biparietal diameter in predicting fetal weight, gestational age, and the time of onset of spontaneous labor. We feel that up to the 33rd week of gestation the BPD predicts the age of the fetus with reasonable accuracy; and, therefore, because age and weight are closely related up to that time, it also predicts weight. After the 33rd week there is only a loose association between BPD and weight.

The biparietal diameter is not the only index of fetal head size, but it is the easiest to measure and has been generally accepted. The occipital frontal diameter may also be measured, and formulas are available relating it to fetal weight and maturity (see Appendix). Garrett and Robinson use the cross-sectional area of the fetal skull as their index of the maturity after 28 weeks (see Appendix). This method, since it integrates a large number of diameters, is statistically superior to biparietal diameter measurement but is unfortunately beyond the capability of most clinical laboratories at present. It would be very useful if manufacturers were to include in their machines devices for electronically computing area measurements. These could be used to facilitate the measurement of the area of the fetal head, thorax, or abdomen. A detailed description of these measurements will be presented in Chapter 6 on "Abnormal Growth and Development."

We have discussed the advantages and limitations of the biparietal measurement, but we have not as yet discussed the proper method of measuring the biparietal diameter. First of all, the fetal presentation must be known and is most rapidly obtained by means of real-time scanning. Assuming that the fetus is in a vertex presentation and that the position of the head is occiput transverse, a sagittal scan will produce a coronal section through the fetal head. The falx lies at the top of this coronal section, and in the case of a vertex presentation with the head in occiput transverse, it points caudally with respect to the maternal abdomen. One could measure the biparietal diameter at the level of the base of the falx. However, it is easier to perform scans at right angles to the sagittal section. Assuming the conditions previously described (occiput transverse), one can now produce a series of fronto-occipital sections through the falx down to the level of the ventricular system. The objective is to obtain the widest of the diameters which contains the midline (falx), and with modern equipment it is possible to identify the ventricular system in this section. As a further check, the

Figure 4a
Standard method of obtaining BPD.
Sagittal scan.

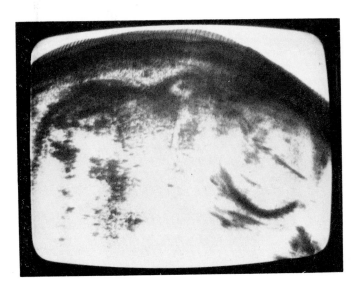

biparietal diameter, as measured in the horizontal cuts, should equal the diameter measured in the sagittal cut.

It has been suggested in the literature that the correct angle for obtaining fronto-occipital sections of the fetal head is 90° from the coronal section. This is true if the head has not moved in the interim; unfortunately, it frequently does.

If the fetal head is in an occiput transverse position, horizontal scans made at right angles to the angle of the fetal head, which has been determined from the sagittal scan, will produce a series of ovoid-shaped sections. When these pass through the falx, the midline echo will extend from the front to the back of the ovoid fronto-occipital section (Figures 4a and 4b). *Finding a symmetrically-placed midline running across an ovoid section does not insure that one has obtained the widest or true biparietal diameter.* The sections which are higher in the fetal head will also contain a complete midline echo (Figure 5). Therefore, it is important to make multiple sections and select the section which has the widest diameter. This maneuver is relatively easy to perform using real-time equipment in which the transducer head can be moved up and down and the images observed as

Figure 4b

BPD when fetus is in occiput transverse position.
Transverse scan.Leading edge to leading edge.
Outside to inside.

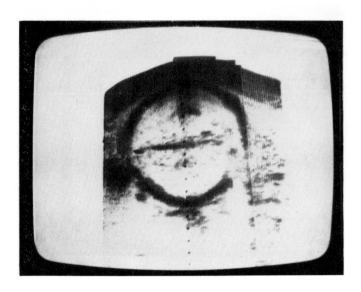

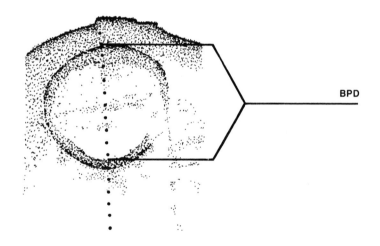

BPD

Figure 5

Transverse cuts through fetal head, each productive of a physiological midline.

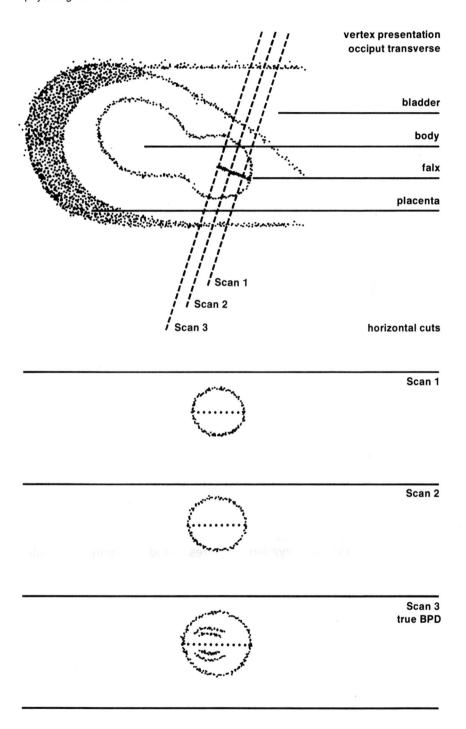

these motions are performed. With contact scanners, it is necessary to develop a technique which simulates that of the real-time scanner. That is, the operator must make rapid motions, moving the scanner arm very slightly with each motion until the optimal diameter has been obtained. The fetal head may be quite mobile, and its position may be changing from occiput transverse to occiput oblique. Under those circumstances, real-time equipment becomes indispensable.

If the section which has been obtained is not ovoid but circular in shape and contains only the falx or ventricular echoes, one is dealing with a suboccipitobregmatic section. If the skull echograms contain echoes from the floor of the anterior fossa or the temporal bone, the plane is oblique, and an accurate biparietal diameter measurement cannot be made.

It is easiest to obtain the biparietal diameter when the head is in an occiput transverse position. The greater the obliquity of the fetal head, the more difficult it is to obtain a satisfactory biparietal diameter. When the head is markedly oblique, gentle pressure may restore it to a more acceptable position, or the head may be elevated from the pelvis. When the occiput is either directly anterior or posterior, it is impossible to obtain an accurate biparietal measurement. If the fetus is in transverse lie, the method of obtaining the biparietal diameter is exactly the opposite of that outlined for the vertex presentation. The sagittal sections will generally produce the best results. In breech presentation, the proper cut is quite variable and is frequently an oblique section. One must have in mind the desired result, that is, an ovoid section with a complete midline and, if possible, the ventricular system (Figures 6 and 7). (Either the lateral ventricles (Figure 6) or posterior third ventricle (Figure 7) would be good landmarks. The former must not be confused with the Sylvian vessels, which can be seen to pulsate with real-time equipment.) A circular section may also be used but is less desirable.

Some positions of the fetal head simply do not permit a satisfactory biparietal diameter measurement. If the clinical situation is such that an approximation is permissible, this should be obtained; but the report must indicate that the measurement is only an approximation. Engagement of the fetal head also prevents adequate measurement of the biparietal diameter in some cases.

Figure 6

Real-time scan of head with 8 cm. BPD.
Lateral ventricles are demonstrated.

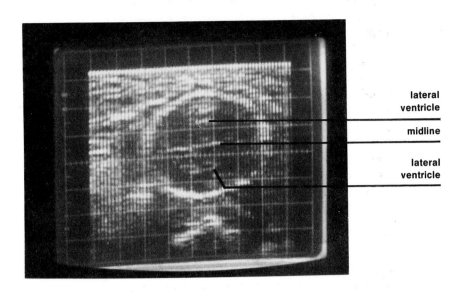

lateral
ventricle

midline

lateral
ventricle

Figure 7

Real-time scan of fetal head showing the midline and posterior
third ventricle. The black shadows on the side are the calipers
placed directly on the oscilloscope.

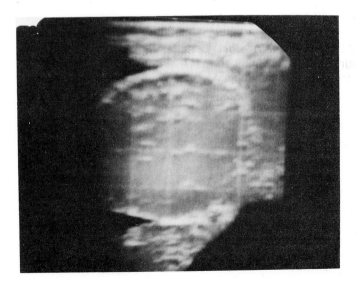

The biparietal diameter may be measured in B-mode or A-mode, but it must be located with B-mode. There are certain theoretical advantages to measuring it in A-mode. The non-uniformity of the cathode ray tube or television screen is not a problem when measurement is made with A-mode. Also comb markers are available which can be expanded. Some commercially available equipment has electronic calipers that can be set at the end points of the measurement. This is advantageous and should be included in equipment used for obstetrical scanning. If a photographic image is being measured, it must be done with a fine caliper; and a photograph of the graticule made from the same camera to oscilloscope distance must be employed. If measurements are made from a television screen, they can only be made from that part of the graticule overlying the fetal head where both graticule and fetal head are identically distorted.

It should be pointed out that the methods used by different investigators to measure biparietal diameter are not identical. Most measurements of BPD are made from leading edge to leading edge. Anatomically, this means that one is measuring from the skin of the proximal side of the fetal head to the inner table of the distal side of the fetal skull. Some workers use signal processing either in an A- or B-mode which does not cut out the distal scalp; that is, they measure from the leading edge on the proximal side to the falling edge on the distal side. To add to the confusion, some who use leading edge measurements compensate for the scalp thickness as well as for the difference in velocity of sound in bone by calibrating their machines at 1600 m./sec. rather than at 1540 m./sec. (a difference of almost 4% which results in the addition of about 3.5 mm. in the full-term fetal head). We feel that this "correction" compensates for two different problems in one imprecise way; that is, it makes all other measurements performed on the same machine 4% too large, and it ignores the fact that the thickness of the fetal skull is variable. For clinical purposes, however, absolute accuracy of measurement is not crucial as long as the method employed is consistent and the numbers have meaning in the laboratory in which they are used. In our appendix we include tables of leading edge to leading edge and leading edge of falling edge.

In summary, the biparietal diameter, if carefully measured, is an accurate means of dating a pregnancy in the second and early third trimesters. Biparietal diameters of 8.5 cm. and above do not show a close correlation with the length of gestation. In the late third trimester, the rate of growth of the fetal head is slow, and the standard error of measurement may be equal to or greater than 1 week's growth. Thus, we recommend that biparietal diameter measurements be made as early in the pregnancy as possible for dating. A series of readings is preferable to a single reading since it provides a further check on the accuracy of the single reading and gives useful information about the rate of growth of the fetus. The patient may be in doubt about the date of her last menstrual period, but the time elapsed between ultrasonic measurements is never in doubt. The biparietal diameter is a relatively insensitive method of assessing growth retardation, and other methods which will be discussed in a later chapter should be used for that purpose.

References

1 **Bergsjoo, P., Bakke, T., and Salamonsen, L.** Observer error in ultrasonic fetal cephalometry. Acta Obstet. Gynecol. Scand. 54:41, 1975.

2 **Campbell, S.** An improved method of fetal cephalometry by ultrasound. Obstet. Gynaecol. Br. Commonw. 75:568, 1968.

3 **Campbell, S.** Ultrasonic fetal cephalometry during the second trimester of pregnancy. J. Obstet. Gynaecol. Br. Commonw. 77:1057, 1970.

4 **Davison, J.M., Lind, T., Farr, V., and Whittingham, T.A.** The limitations of ultrasonic fetal cephalometry. J. Obstet. Gynaecol. Br. Commonw. 80:769, 1973.

5 **Garrett, W.J., and Robinson, D.E.** Assessment of fetal size and growth rate by ultrasonic echoscopy. Obstet. Gynecol. 38:525, 1971.

6 **Goldstein, P., Gershenson, D., and Hobbins, J. C.** Fetal biparietal diameter as a predictor of a mature lecithin sphingomyelin ratio. Obstet. Gynecol. 48:667, 1976.

7 **Ianniruberto, A., and Gibbons, J.M., Jr.** Predicting fetal weight by ultrasonic B-scan cephalometry. An improved technic with disappointing results. Obstet. Gynecol. 37:689, 1971.

8 **Lee, B.O., Major, F.J., and Weingold, A.B.** Ultrasonic determination of fetal maturity at repeat cesarean section. Obstet. Gynecol. 38:294, 1971.

9 **Levi, S.** Ultrasonic diagnosis in obstetrics. Clinical value of measuring the biparietal diameter of the fetus. Gynecol. Obstet. (Paris) 69:227, 1970.

10 **Levi, S., and Erbsman, F.** Antenatal fetal growth from the nineteenth week. Ultrasonic study of 12 head and chest dimensions. Am. J. Obstet. Gynecol. 121:262, 1975.

11 **Lunt, R.M., and Chard, T.** Reproducibility of measurement of fetal biparietal diameter by ultrasonic cephalometry. J. Obstet. Gynaecol. Br. Commonw. 81:682, 1974.

12 **Robinson, H.P.** Gestation sac: volumes as determined by sonar in the first trimester of pregnancy. Br. J. Obstet. Gynaecol. 82:100, 1975.

13 **Robinson, H.P.** Sonar measurement of fetal crown-rump length as means of assessing maturity in first trimester of pregnancy. Br. Med. J. 4:28, 1973.

14 **Sabbagha, R.E., Turner, J.H., Rockette, H., Mazer, J., and Orgill, J.** Sonar BPD and fetal age. Definition of the relationship. Obstet. Gynecol. 43:7, 1974.

15 **Sanders, R.C.** Letter: Fetal biparietal diameters correlated with gestational age. J. Clin. Ultrasound 1:344, 1973.

16 **Varma, T.R.** Prediction of delivery date by ultrasound cephalometry. J. Obstet. Gynaecol. Br. Commonw. 80:316, 1973.

17 **Watmough, D.** A critical assessment of ultrasonic foetal cephalometry. Br. J. Radiol. 46:566, 1973.

The Placenta

4

The identification of the placenta and the changes which occur in it with maturation and disease requires equipment with wide dynamic range (gray scale). In writings about the placenta which appeared in the late sixties, there is little mentioned about the texture of the placenta or the changes produced by disease. The exceptions to this are some articles in the German literature by workers using real-time equipment and in the English literature by Australians using gray scale instruments. Placental texture was not initially appreciated because of the use of leading edge bistable scanning. The placenta is an organ containing a complex parenchymal structure, very much like the liver. In order to appreciate its texture, echoes from small structures must be represented, and this requires wide dynamic range.

In an earlier chapter, we stressed the importance of a full bladder for visualization of the uterus. This is also true for visualization of the uterine cervix and low-lying placentas. Placenta previa cannot be accurately diagnosed unless the bladder is full enough so that the lower uterine segment can be seen. Before discussing the use of B-scan, the Doppler method of placental localization should be mentioned briefly. Although it may be possible to determine whether a placenta is anterior or posterior using the Doppler technique, the diagnosis of placenta previa cannot be reliably made. Furthermore, it is rarely of clinical value to know on which wall the placenta is implanted. Knowing that the placenta is posteriorly located does not define the best place for amniocentesis, nor does the existence of an anterior placenta exclude amniocentesis. In our opinion, therefore, the Doppler method of localizing the placenta has little clinical value and should not be employed.

In the older ultrasound literature, 95% accuracy was claimed for placental localization. With modern equipment, the accuracy of localization should be effectively 100%. The placenta is readily identified by its juxtaposition with the amniotic fluid, as well as by its appearance. The mid-trimester placenta has a relatively homogeneous parenchymal texture except for the chorionic plate which lies in contact with the amniotic cavity. The interface between amniotic cavity and chorionic plate is a strong one, accentuated by the fibrous tissue just beneath the chorionic plate; thus, it is recognized as a dark line (Figure 1). No problem should be encountered in finding an anterior placenta unless the gain controls are manipulated in such a way that its echoes are suppressed. Reverberations from the abdominal wall can be confused with the placenta. However, their appearance is different in that they exactly parallel the contour of the abdominal wall, and they do not have the texture of placenta. Similar reverberating echoes can be seen from any fluid-containing structure including the urinary bladder. When the bladder and the uterus are scanned together, the reverberating echoes are seen to continue from the uterus into the bladder.

The posterior placenta does not differ acoustically from the anterior placenta. It may differ in appearance, however, because the sonic beam can be attenuated by intervening fetal parts. When no interference is created by intervening parts, it looks exactly the same as an anterior placenta. Unless there is almost no amniotic fluid, some portion of the posterior placenta can always be identified. This is best done by scanning lateral to the fetus. When one has real-time equipment, the moving fetus can be seen to cast shadows on the posterior placenta (Figure 2), and different portions of it will be noted to come in and out of view as other portions are eclipsed by the intervening fetal parts. When the placenta is shadowed by fetal parts, the posterior uterine wall, because of its stronger interface, is still visible at high gain settings. The pulsating echoes of the aorta or iliac arteries beneath the uterus can often be seen with real-time equipment.

Figure 1

Anterior placenta.
Sagittal scan through fetal limbs.

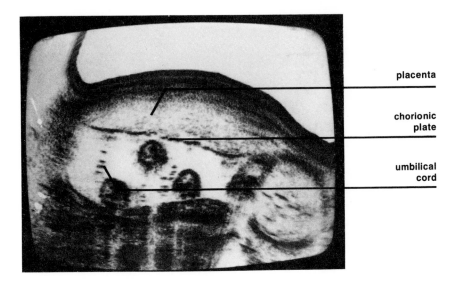

placenta

chorionic
plate

umbilical
cord

Figure 2

Real-time representation of acoustic shadowing by fetal small
parts.

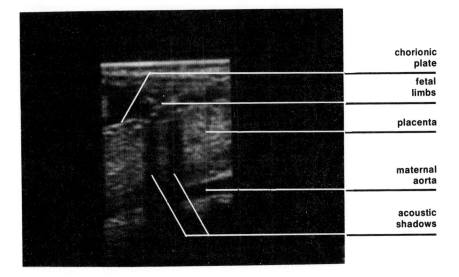

chorionic
plate

fetal
limbs

placenta

maternal
aorta

acoustic
shadows

Figure 3

Marginal anterior placenta previa proven at cesarean section.

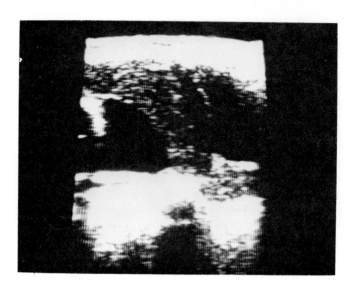

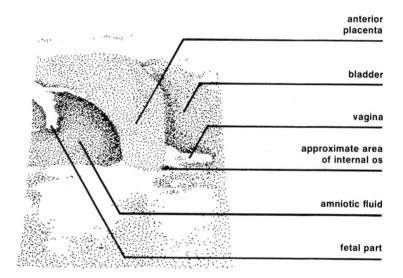

anterior placenta

bladder

vagina

approximate area of internal os

amniotic fluid

fetal part

Although the localization of the placenta can be made with 100% accuracy, the determination of whether it crosses the cervix is slightly less accurate. This is due to the impossibility of precisely localizing the internal os of the cervix (Figure 3). Because of this problem, one occasionally encounters a case in which the placenta is felt to be most likely marginally previa, but the diagnosis cannot be made with certainty.

Before ultrasonic localization of the placenta was routinely practiced, it was not appreciated that its relationship to the cervix changes as the pregnancy progresses. Therefore, it was considered that the diagnosis of placenta previa necessarily required that the patient be delivered by cesarean section (Figures 4 and 5). We now know that it is quite common in the second and occasionally in the third trimester to find a placenta which covers the cervix and later find that it no longer occupies that position. It is difficult to explain physiologically this fortunate change of position in cases of central placenta previa, but apparently there is lengthening of the lower uterine segment, with displacement away from the cervix. One of three possibilities can occur in a patient with placenta previa who presents with bleeding during the second trimester:

1 Bleeding will cease and the patient will eventually be delivered vaginally.
2 The patient will bleed acutely and require emergency cesarean section.
3 The patient will remain with a placenta previa until term and then require cesarean section.

Unfortunately, there is no way to predict into which of these three categories an individual patient will fall.

Statistically, the overwhelming majority of the patients who have placenta previa in the second trimester, even those who are symptomatic, will do well. But since patients cannot be treated as statistics, it is mandatory to take necessary precautions and repeat the ultrasonic examination at 2-week intervals until the position of the placenta is normal or the fetus is full-term, whichever occurs first. If, as often happens, placenta previa is discovered as an incidental finding in the course of an examination for some other reason and the patient is symptomatic, we advocate follow-up examinations at 2-week intervals if a large volume of placenta crosses the cervix. If only a small tongue of placenta crosses the cervix in the second trimester and the patient is asymptomatic, it is virtually certain that the placenta will be in normal position at term.

Figure 4

Experience with ultrasonic diagnosis of 42 cases of placenta previa
at Montreal General Hospital in 1971–1972.

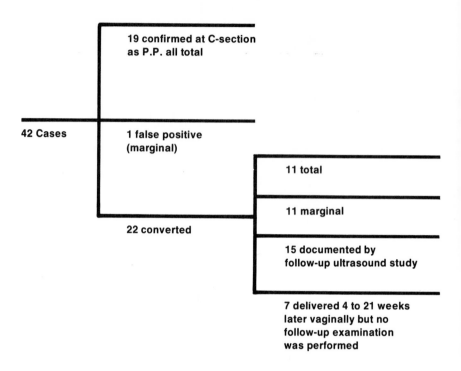

*Under no circumstances should the diagnosis of
placenta previa, made more than 2 weeks prior to the
time of delivery, be used as the basis for **elective**
cesarean section.* The ultrasonic study must be
repeated since the position of the placenta with
respect to the cervix may change even as late as the
38th week.

Since no difficulty is encountered in identifying an
anterior placenta, when an anterior placenta crosses
the cervix this is relatively easy to see. Difficulty arises
when there is a posterior placenta previa with a vertex
presentation because the posterior placenta is
shadowed by the fetal head, and one sees a clear
space between the fetal·head and the posterior
uterine wall, rather than the placenta behind the fetal
head (Figure 6).

However, if the bladder is full, a segment of placenta
which lies inferior to the fetal head can be identified.
As one scans up from the cervix, one sees
successively the placenta beneath the urinary
bladder, a fetal head which is separated from the
uterine wall by a clear space (the eclipsed placenta),
and finally the posterior placenta which lies above the

Figure 5

Experience with placenta previa at Montreal General Hospital 1971–1972, expressed as function of gestational age at the time the diagnosis was made.

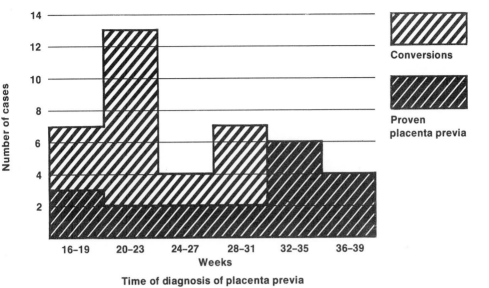

Time of diagnosis of placenta previa

fetal shadow (Figure 7). If pressure is applied to the fetal head, the distance between it and the posterior uterine wall does not change; however, if there is no placenta between the fetal head and the uterine wall, the fetal head can be depressed so that it touches the posterior uterine wall. Another maneuver which is useful in suspected posterior placenta previa is to place the patient in Trendelenburg position. This may move the head out of the pelvis and permits visualization of the posterior placenta previa. A step-like configuration of the placenta may be observed as it crosses the cervix.

With experience there should be no difficulty in identifying posterior placenta previa if the problem of shadowing of the posterior placenta by the fetal head is kept in mind. When the fetus is in breech or transverse position, there are usually fetal limbs moving about in the region of the cervix. Since the placenta is a barrier to the motion of the limbs, if the limbs can be seen to move into the cervix, the diagnosis of placenta previa can be excluded. Otherwise, one sees the limbs abutting against the placenta, and one identifies the placenta as it is alternately visible and invisible depending upon the position of the fetal limbs.

Figure 6

Schematic illustration of findings in posterior placenta previa when transverse scans are performed at levels 1 and 2.

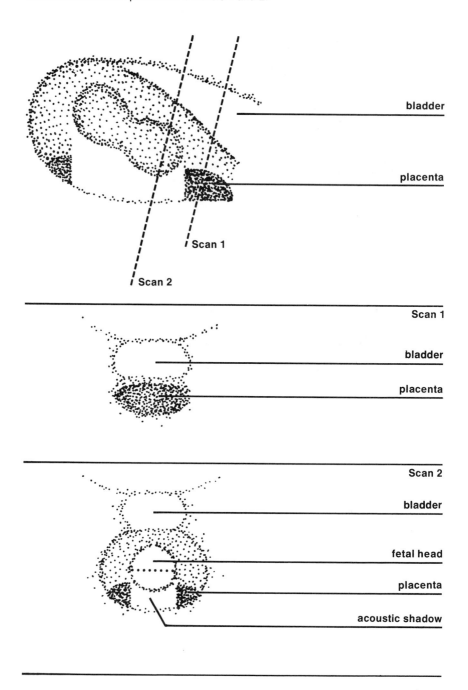

bladder

placenta

Scan 1

Scan 2

Scan 1

bladder

placenta

Scan 2

bladder

fetal head

placenta

acoustic shadow

Figure 7

Scans at different levels in placenta previa.

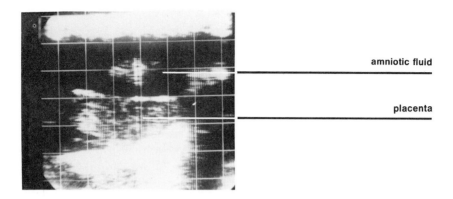

amniotic fluid

placenta

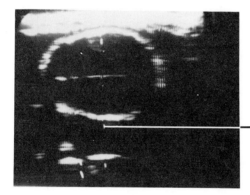

clear space
representing placenta

The only limitation to the accuracy of the diagnosis of placenta previa is the identification of the cervix. When the bladder is full, the cervix can be assumed to lie at the point where the bladder-uterus interface intersects with the posterior vaginal wall. However, as shown in the work of Sanders, the internal os may lie slightly above that point, so that in some cases one cannot be sure whether the position of the placenta is normal or a marginal previa is present. To decide how to manage the patient with suspected placenta previa at term, we advocate the following strategy:

1   If placenta previa has been excluded without doubt by ultrasonic examination, there is no need to do a vaginal examination.
2   If, on the other hand, a placenta previa has been diagnosed with certainty, a vaginal examination is not indicated and may be dangerous.

3   In a case when it is not certain whether there is a
     marginal placenta previa or a placenta which does
     not cross the cervix, a "double set-up" exam
     should be performed before delivery. However,
     we have found that with increasing experience,
     these cases are rare.

Volumetric measurements of the placenta have been
made, and these are useful in pointing to the
possibilities of certain pathological states such as
diabetes, rhesus incompatibility, and placental
insufficiency. Generally, the experienced
ultrasonographer can "eyeball" the volume of the
placenta with reasonable accuracy. As we learn more
about the effects of different diseases on the
placenta, we are now able to correlate these effects
with morphological findings demonstrated by
ultrasound. For example, diabetic mothers have a
tendency to deliver macrosomic infants. Since the
placenta is a fetal organ, it is also affected by the
macrosomic stimulation. With severe diabetes, small
vessel disease may result in a shrunken placenta.
When there is placental insufficiency, the volume of
the placenta is small, and the amount of amniotic
fluid is also relatively small. The uterus appears to be
crowded with fetal parts and placenta.

In the normal gestation, the cotyledons become
visible at about 36 weeks. Since they are engorged
with blood, they appear to be relatively transonic
whereas the intercotyledonous septa are sono-
reflective. The mature placenta with visible
cotyledonous structure has the appearance of Swiss
cheese (Figure 8). Often the multi-textured
appearance can best be appreciated in white on black
(Figures 9a and 9b). Since the diseased placenta is
very much like the senile placenta, when there is
pre-eclampsia a mature-appearing placenta may be
seen before 36 weeks and indicates the presence of a
pathological pregnancy (Figure 10). Although the
mature placenta almost always contains multiple
small foci of calcification, the ring-like echoes
observed in the placenta are not necessarily
produced by calcium since the distribution of
calcium in the placenta is frequently generalized and
has no specific architecture.

Figure 8

Real-time scan of mature placenta.
Note texture.

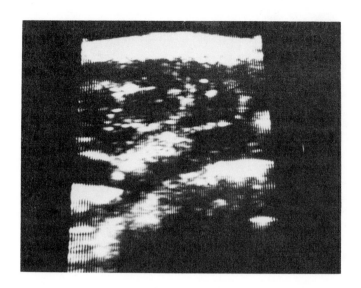

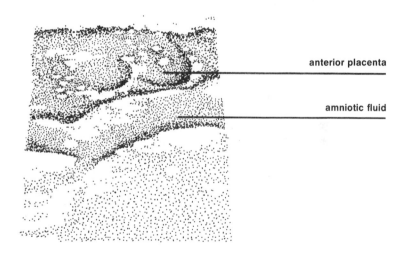

anterior placenta

amniotic fluid

Figure 9a

Mature placenta in gray scale black on white.

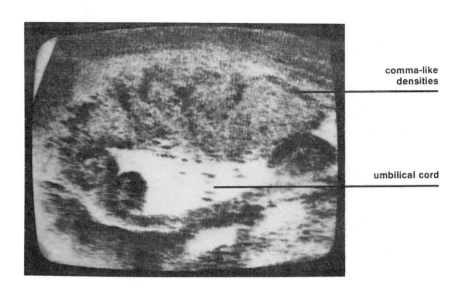

comma-like
densities

umbilical cord

Figure 9b

Same mature placenta with white on black "swiss cheese" texture
easily appreciated.

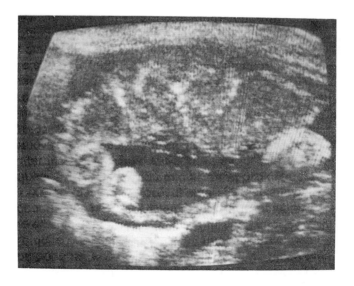

Figure 10

Mature appearing placenta in toxemic patient at 34 weeks.

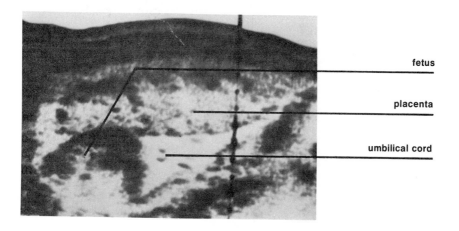

fetus

placenta

umbilical cord

In rhesus incompatibility, the placenta is edematous, and the solid elements are separated by fluid. In addition, the placenta is thicker than normal. The thickness, in fact, may be correlated with the severity of the disease. In hydrops, the placental thickness is more than 5 cm., and the solid elements are separated by edema (Figure 11).

Isolated mucinous cysts are seen in the placenta, and mucinous degeneration of the choroid can be identified ultrasonically (Figure 12). These are generally benign conditions.

Placental infarction is common in late pregnancy and also produces textural changes in the placenta (Figure 13). When there are relatively small amounts of retroplacental bleeding, the blood accumulates under the membranes in the lower uterus (Figure 14). The placenta is not displaced away from the uterine wall by a collection of blood unless the bleeding is massive (Figure 15). The demonstration of blood elevating the membranes, which we believe to be a finding of retroplacental bleeding, can be compatible with normal progression of the pregnancy.

Figure 11
Real-time scans of hydropic anterior placenta.

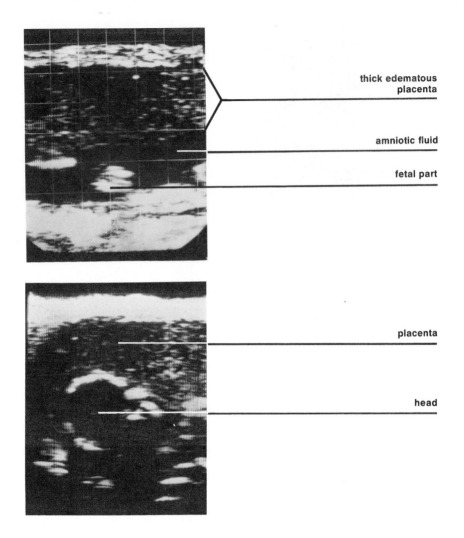

thick edematous placenta

amniotic fluid

fetal part

placenta

head

Figure 12
Mucinous degeneration of choroid.

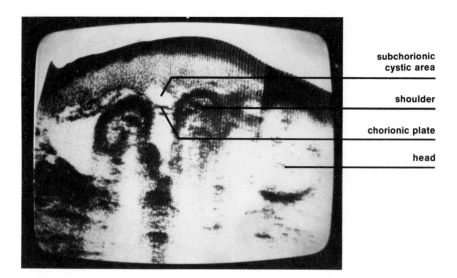

subchorionic
cystic area

shoulder

chorionic plate

head

In the early second trimester, there may be an apparent separation of the uterine wall from the placenta. We believe that the most likely explanation for this phenomenon is that there is residual compact decidua (decidua basalis) between the placenta and uterus. In any case, these pregnancies have a normal prognosis, and subsequent examinations will show normal contact between the placenta and uterine wall (Figure 16).

The study of morphological abnormalities of the placenta has received too little attention in the past because of deficiencies in equipment. We hope that more attention will be devoted to this problem in the future since it may provide an important means of early diagnosis of intrauterine deprivation.

Figure 13
Magnified view of infarcted posterior fundal placenta.

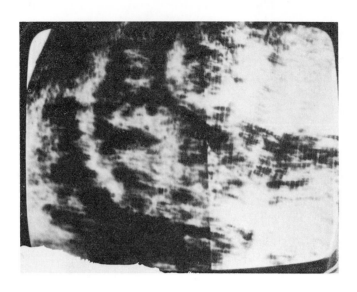

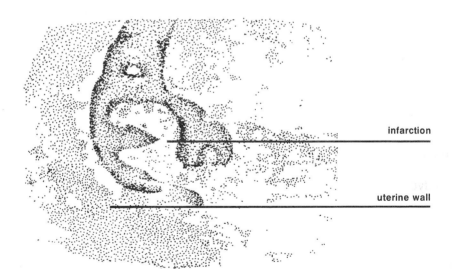

Figure 14

Placental separation in midtrimester gestation.
Note elevation of membranes posteriorly by blood clot dissecting
around laterally from anterior placenta.

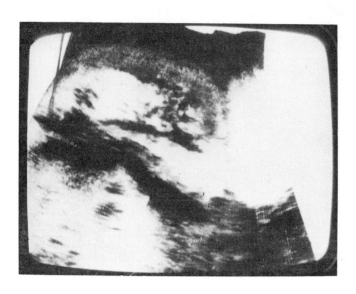

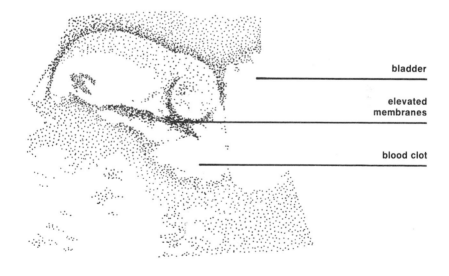

bladder

elevated
membranes

blood clot

Figure 15

Magnified scan of patient requiring emergency cesarean section
for abruption involving one-third of placental surface.

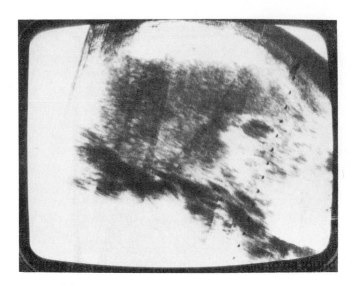

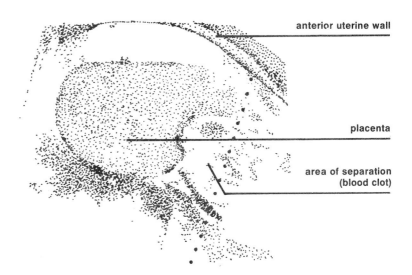

anterior uterine wall

placenta

area of separation
(blood clot)

Figure 16

Real-time scan of apparent displacement of posterior placenta in subsequently normal second trimester pregnancy.

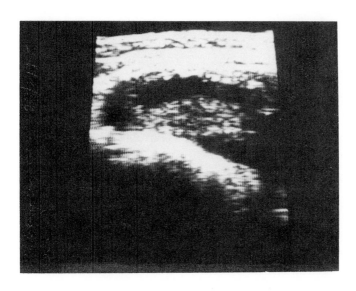

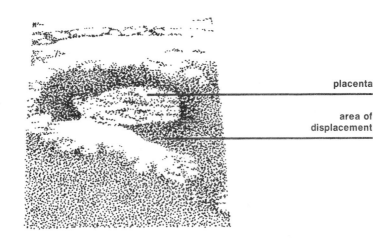

placenta

area of
displacement

References

1   **Donald, I.** Proceedings: placental localization by sonar — a safe procedure. Br. J. Radiol. 47:72, 1974.

2   **Gottesfeld, K.R., Thompson, H.E., Holmes, J.H., and Taylor, E.S.** Ultrasonic placentography — a new method for placental localization. Am. J. Obstet. Gynecol. 96:538, 1966.

3   **Herschlein, H.J.** Diagnosis of abruptio placentae in normally located placentae by means of ultrasonic technique. Aerztl. Forsch. 24:210, 1970.

4   **Holländer, H.J., and Mast, H.** Ultrasonic measurement of the placental thickness in normal pregnancies and Rh incompatibility. Geburtshilfe Frauenheilkd. 28:662, 1968.

5   **Karimi, R.** Failure to diagnose placenta praevia by ultrasound. Lancet 1:1242, 1971.

6   **King, D.L.** Placenta migration demonstrated by ultrasonography. A hypothesis of dynamic placentation. Radiology 109:167, 1973.

7   **Kobayashi, M., Hellman, L.M., and Fillisti, L.** Placental localization by ultrasound. Am. J. Obstet. Gynecol. 106:279, 1970.

8   **Reed, M.F.** Ultrasonic placentography. Br. J. Radiol. 46:255, 1973.

9   **Robinson, D.E., and Garrett, W.J.** Ultrasonic visualization of the placenta. Med. J. Aust. 2:1062, 1970.

10 **Sanders, R.C.** Localization of the cervix in ultrasonic placentography with the use of a fluid-filled pessary. Am. J. Obstet. Gynecol. 118:566, 1974.

11 **Varma, T.R.** Fetal growth and placental function in patients with placenta praevia. J. Obstet. Gynaecol. Br. Commonw. 80:311, 1973.

12 **Winsberg, F.** Echographic changes with placental aging. J. Clin. Ultrasound 1:52, 1973.

Late Pregnancy

5

In other sections we have covered the most common reasons why physicians request ultrasound examinations which include dating the pregnancy, monitoring fetal growth, and localizing the placenta. In late gestation, however, there are a variety of other questions asked of the ultrasonographer stemming from the physician's clinical suspicion that something is amiss with the pregnancy. The reasons for referral would include a large- or small-for-dates uterus, a suspicion of fetal death, a clinical appreciation of an abnormal fetal presentation, or complicating conditions such as Rh disease and diabetes.

Multiple gestation

If we were to use last menstrual period alone for pregnancy dating, the most common reason for a large-for-dates uterus would be that the patient's dates were incorrect. The second most likely possibility would be the presence of a multiple gestation. The diagnosis of multiple pregnancy depends upon the identification of multiple fetuses. There are two major pitfalls to be avoided. A false diagnosis of twins can be made if the fetal head and thorax are both thought to be fetal heads. Because of the smooth ovoid outline of the breech in the second trimester, this may also be mistaken for a fetal head. There are numerous ways to avoid this error. The well-defined borders of the fetal head and the identification of the midline should distinguish it from the thorax or breech even where real-time equipment is not available (Figure 1). In addition, by tracing along the fetal spine, one can distinguish the head from the breech, and the fetal thorax and head can be seen to merge. When real-time equipment is available, a fetal thorax is easily identified since it contains the pulsating fetal heart.

Figure 1
Fetal head and trunk of mid-trimester fetus.

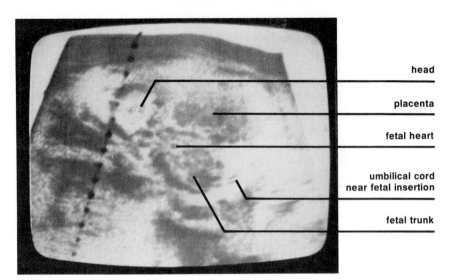

head

placenta

fetal heart

umbilical cord
near fetal insertion

fetal trunk

The other pitfall is one of omission, that is, missing the multiple gestation. If two circular structures are identified which are separated from each other in a fashion such that they could not possibly belong to the same fetus, it does not matter what those structures are. Therefore, the identification of two such circles should immediately alert one to the presence of twins, and then one must piece together the puzzle. The fetal heads must be related to the corresponding fetal bodies, and the presentation of both fetuses is determined. This is relatively easy to do using real-time equipment (Figures 2a and 2b).

In 5 years' experience with real-time equipment, the only instance in which a multiple pregnancy was missed was in a case in which both fetuses were dead and the heads and bodies were grossly deformed. With similar experience in compound contact scanning, occasionally we have missed twins on routine examination in the second trimester when the diagnosis was not suspected clinically. Irrespective of what method is used, one should develop some means of rapidly scanning the uterus in a systematic way so as to be sure that multiple gestations are not overlooked.

Figure 2a

Twins in vertex, breech presentation.
Sagittal scan in gray scale.

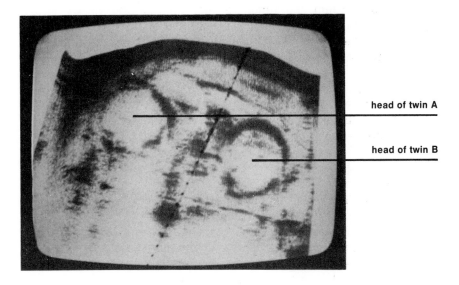

head of twin A

head of twin B

Figure 2b

Real-time scan of twins.

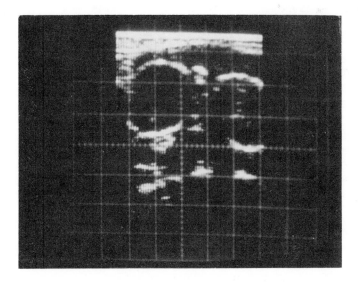

With twins, there may be one or two placentas. It is often difficult to obtain both biparietal diameters since both heads are so mobile. However, when both measurements are obtained, there should be no more than a 3-mm. difference between them. If one wishes to date the pregnancy, the biparietal diameters up until the 33rd week of gestation should be no smaller than those from singleton pregnancies.

Occasionally, monozygotic twins share the same blood supply, resulting in a twin-to-twin transfusion. The fetal arteries or veins may communicate with one another on the fetal surface of the placenta. A serious problem occurs when fetal cotyledons are supplied by arterioles from one twin, and the venules draining those cotyledons convey the blood back to the other twin. This would mean that a small amount of essential blood volume would be depleted from the donor twin with each beat of its heart. If the donor twin is severely affected, it may die in the late second trimester or early third trimester. The recipient may also die due to cardiac overload. If the condition is not lethal to either twin, there is a marked discrepancy at the time of birth between the plethoric recipient twin and the scrawny, growth-retarded donor. The diagnosis is conclusively made when there is a difference in infant weight of more than 30%. Both twins require immediate and aggressive management in a newborn special care unit; therefore, it is extremely important to make this diagnosis in utero as early as possible. One can suspect the diagnosis when there is a discrepancy of more than 2 weeks between the twin biparietal diameter measurements. Trunk measurements are also extremely valuable in predicting a disparity in fetal weights. Since the blood volume of the recipient twin is often increased, the fetal renal plasma flow may be appreciably enhanced, resulting in the production of copious amounts of urine. This frequently leads to polyhydramnios. Urine production rates, discussed in another chapter, are useful in this condition when it is possible to obtain these measurements. As the gestation progresses, serial scans will demonstrate an augmented discrepancy in the dimensions between twins. In these cases, the in utero diagnosis of a twin-to-twin transfusion could save the life of either twin if delivery could be accomplished at survivable gestations.

We have recently made the diagnosis of fetal death in a donor twin 4 weeks after noting a discrepancy between biparietal diameters. Fetal death resulted in the development of disseminated intravascular coagulation (DIC) in the mother. The recipient twin, however, was spared from this coagulopathy because the vascular communication in the placenta was closed off by thrombosis in the communicating vessels.

In most cases, twins mature pulmonically at the same time of gestation, but there are reports of discrepancies between L/S ratios in twins. If one wishes to obtain information about the condition and maturity of each twin by amniocentesis, it is necessary to tap both sacs. This would be an extremely difficult undertaking without ultrasound, but with gray scale imaging one can clearly discern the separating membranes, and appropriate sites for amniocentesis are chosen with this information. We suggest that a small amount of dye such as indigo carmen be injected after the fluid is withdrawn from the first sac. If dye is found in the fluid obtained during the second amniocentesis, this would indicate that the same sac has been entered twice.

Locking of twins is extremely rare. The prerequisite for this unfortunate mechanical phenomenon occurs when the first twin, twin A, presents as a breech, and twin B is a vertex. The small parts overlap in the midline. During the delivery of the breech, the aftercoming head becomes obstructed by the vertex of twin B. It is important to alert the referring physician to this possibility, since cesarean section may be indicated.

Figure 3

Breech presentation.

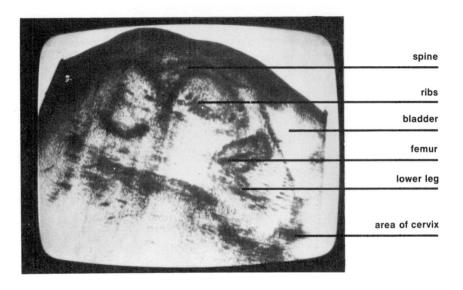

spine

ribs

bladder

femur

lower leg

area of cervix

Figure 4

Transverse scan of fetus in transverse lie.
Note fetal bladder.

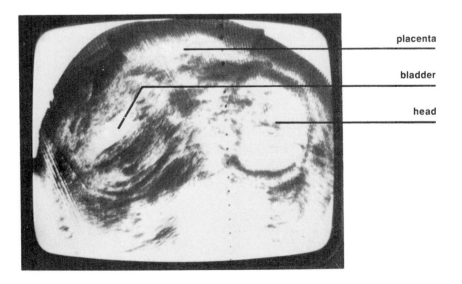

placenta

bladder

head

Breech presentation

With ultrasound one can unerringly diagnose whether a fetus is in a breech presentation (Figure 3), a vertex presentation, or a transverse lie (Figure 4); however, in an obese woman it is difficult to determine clinically the presentation of a fetus. At term, approximately 4% of patients present with babies in the breech presentation. At about 32 weeks, however, 8–10% of babies are in a breech presentation. Because babies born by breech delivery are subject to higher rates of morbidity and mortality, some physicians will attempt to convert breeches into a more favorable position by external version. If the pregnancy is far from term, the majority of these babies will spontaneously return to their original position. The likelihood of permanent success is greater between 33 and 37 weeks. With ultrasound, it is possible to determine the position of the fetus before, during, and after external version.

Ultrasound is extremely useful in the management of patients in labor with breech presentations because it is necessary to know the exact size of the fetal head, and x-ray pelvimetry cannot provide sufficiently accurate information about head size. Since a cord can prolapse following rupture of membranes in a footling breech, it is desirable to have an ultrasound machine convenient to the delivery floor in the event that this obstetrical emergency occurs during scanning.

Although today roentgen pelvimetry is being utilized less frequently, this diagnostic modality remains essential in primiparas with breech presentations; and on the university service at Yale, pelvimetry is performed on *all* patients in labor with breeches. If any measurement of the pelvis is borderline, a cesarean section is performed.

Since most of the fetal morbidity in breeches is a result of traumatic delivery of the aftercoming head, we feel that if the biparietal diameter is above 9.6 cm. (leading edge), the baby should be delivered by cesarean section regardless of the maternal pelvic measurements. If the biparietal diameter is between 9.3 and 9.6, vaginal delivery should be attempted only through a capacious pelvis, especially in a primipara breech.

Another indication for cesarean section is the finding of an extended head on x-ray (which may also be suspected ultrasonically). Most obstetricians will empirically perform a cesarean section on these patients to avoid the increased incidence of fetal spinal cord transection.

Prolapse of the umbilical cord is 20 times more common in patients whose babies present as footling breeches because there is incomplete filling of the pelvis by the descending presenting part. It is feasible with gray scale or real-time to scrutinize the contents of the lower uterine segment for the presence of umbilical cord once the patient is in labor. If the cord is found at the level of the buttocks or below, it would be an error for the obstetrician to rupture membranes at this point, and it is the opinion of one author that cesarean section should be performed in the face of this finding.

Fetal death

Missed abortion and fetal death are among those conditions where the patients present as small-for-dates. When there is a missed abortion, the diagnosis is not difficult. No recognizable fetus is present.

Much has been written about the echographic appearance of the dead fetus. While there is no doubt that the diagnosis of a dead fetus can be made when one observes a marked deformity of the fetal skull or body or a bizarre position of the fetus, these are all relatively late findings and do not precede the corresponding radiological findings (Figure 5). The most reliable and easiest finding is the absence of a fetal heart beat, and the best way to detect this absence with reliability is to use real-time scanning. However, having located the fetal thorax, one can also use M-mode or the Doppler technique to demonstrate the fetal heart. Real-time scanning has been 100% reliable in the diagnosis of fetal death. Having established the diagnosis by ultrasound, we generally obtain a radiograph of the abdomen in order to visualize a fetal deformity or anomaly. As was mentioned earlier, the biological tests for pregnancy may remain positive for weeks after missed abortion, incomplete abortion, and fetal death.

Figure 5
Real-time scan of flattened head in fetal demise.

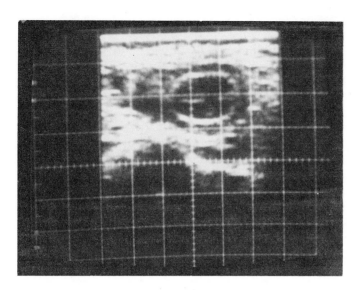

Congenital anomalies and fetal anatomy

The presence of fetal anomalies should be suspected when either excessive or diminished amniotic fluid is noted. Cranial and spinal abnormalities comprise about 10% of all major fetal anomalies. The two most commonly encountered cranial anomalies are anencephaly and hydrocephaly. Women who have already delivered a baby with neural tube defects are subject to a 5% risk that a similar defect will occur in another pregnancy. These patients are now seeking prenatal genetic diagnosis in the second trimester. Amniotic fluid alpha-fetoprotein levels are significantly elevated in most open neural tube defects, including anencephaly. Also, anencephaly can be diagnosed in the second trimester with ultrasound. Using these two modalities together, anencephaly can be predicted with 95% accuracy.

Of babies born with neural tube defects, 95% (1/800 live births in North America) are not predicted in early gestations simply because there is no genetic history to suggest it. Patients with anencephalic fetuses are referred for ultrasound examination because the uterus is large-for-dates. This diagnosis is not difficult to make. The fetal body is easily identified; fetal movements are vigorous and the fetal heart easily found, but a careful search of the uterus shows only a primordial fetal head (Figure 6). It is particularly important to fill a patient's bladder when anencephaly is suspected since the head may be obscured deep in the pelvis. In later gestation, it is prudent to confirm the ultrasonic diagnosis of anencephaly with a radiograph of the abdomen. In the past 5 years using real-time equipment and compound contact scanning, no false positive or false negative diagnoses of anencephaly have been made in the second or third trimester.

Hydrocephaly can be diagnosed ultrasonically in utero by means of two criteria:

1   The fetal head is large for dates with respect to the fetal body (Figure 7a).
2   The fetal ventricular system is enlarged (Figures 7b and 7c).

We indicated in an earlier chapter on fetal biparietal diameter that the ventricular system in the fetus can be identified. The fetal skull, being relatively thin, causes very little attenuation and scattering of ultrasonic beam; thus, it is not surprising that intracranial structures are readily visible. Even in newborn infants it is possible to demonstrate the ventricular system with relatively little difficulty, and the diagnosis of hydrocephalus in infants is made with B-scanning. There are few data concerning sequential measurements of hydrocephalics in early gestation. Abnormal dilatation of the ventricles should precede excessive growth of the biparietal diameter. The fetal skull volume of the hydrocephalic will vary at any time in gestation depending upon the severity of the condition. Data are sparse concerning early changes in biparietal diameter in hydrocephaly, but there is a strong suggestion that in some cases abnormal biparietal diameters are not encountered until late in gestation. There should be no question

Figure 6a
Anencephaly in the second trimester.
Note turtle-like appearance of fetus.

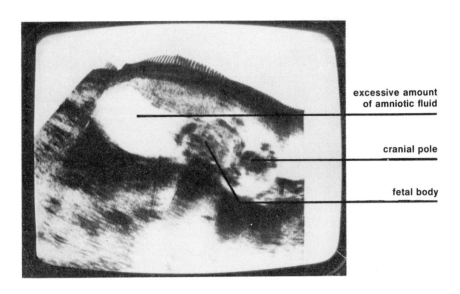

excessive amount
of amniotic fluid

cranial pole

fetal body

Figure 6b
Anencephalic fetus.

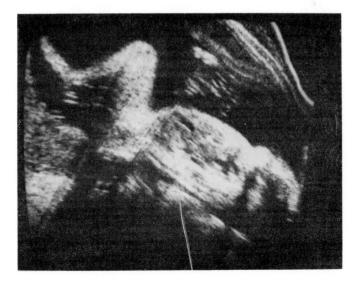

Figure 7a
Sagittal scan of hydrocephalic.

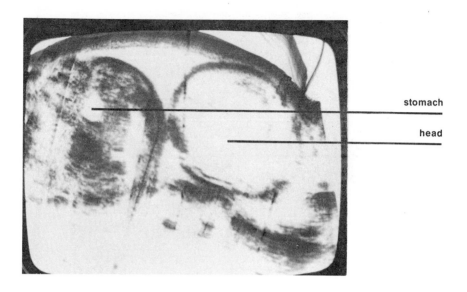

stomach

head

Figure 7b
Ventricular system in 30-week hydrocephalic fetus.

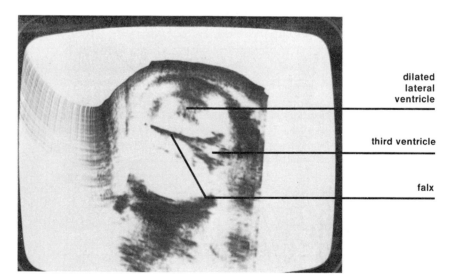

dilated
lateral
ventricle

third ventricle

falx

Figure 7c

Normal ventricular system in 17-week fetus (magnified).

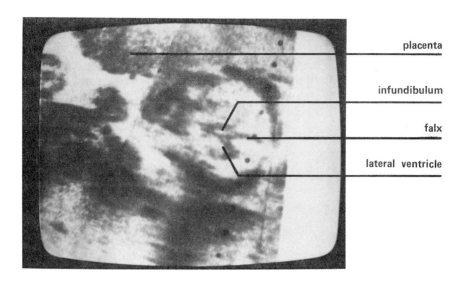

placenta

infundibulum

falx

lateral ventricle

concerning the diagnosis when biparietal diameters are obtained in late gestation in excess of 10.5 cm. On one occasion, we have correctly predicted a porencephalic cyst in utero by noting a shift in the midline structures. Although hydrocephaly is not by strict definition a neural tube defect, 10% of all babies with hydrocephaly also have a spinal defect.

The entire length of the fetal spine can be examined until the 24th week of gestation (Figure 8). After this time, however, the fetal body tucks; and it is extremely difficult with compound contact scanning to see the entire spine on one sagittal scan, although one can easily follow the spinal curve with a real-time scanner. It is definitely feasible to diagnose large spinal defects with newer instruments, but more investigation must be pursued before the accuracy of this method can be assessed, especially in smaller defects (Figure 9).

If oligohydramnios is not present, it is possible to diagnose meningomyelocele. The diagnosis, however, is not easy to make when there is any degree of fetal crowding.

Figure 8

Spine in a 20-week fetus.
Note shadowing from ribs.

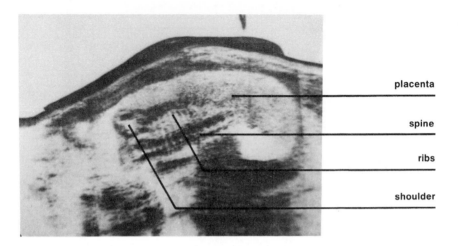

placenta

spine

ribs

shoulder

Figure 9

Apparently normal spine in 18-week fetus who was born with neurologically significant lumbar spina bifida. Amniotic fluid alpha-fetoprotein levels were not significantly elevated.

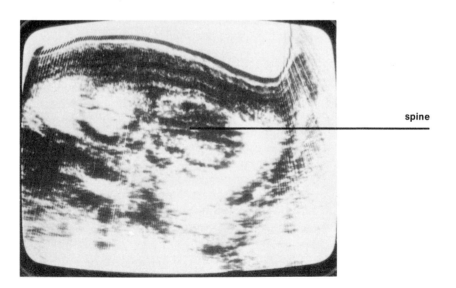

spine

Figure 10a
Real-time scan of fetal aorta.

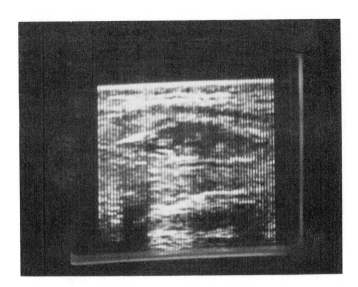

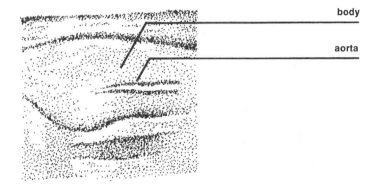

body

aorta

Figure 10b
Fetal inferior vena cava.
Lines displayed are for measurement of total intrauterine volume.

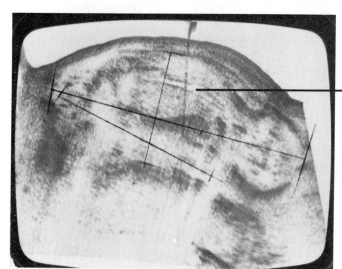

**apparent site of
branching of
inferior vena cava**

As ultrasonic equipment improves, more fetal anatomy can be discerned. Fetal rib cage is identified by a washboard-like pattern of echoes resulting from the penetration of sound between the intercostal spaces (Figure 8). The fetal aorta is visible in front of the fetal spine and is also represented by parallel lines thinner than those produced by the spine. With real-time equipment, the fetal aorta (Figure 10a) can be distinguished from the spine and inferior vena cava (Figure 10b) by the presence of pulsation. As discussed elsewhere, cross sections of the fetus will reveal the umbilical vein (Figure 11) as it enters the liver, which may serve as a good landmark for the measurement of abdominal girth.

The umbilical cord (Figure 12) is represented by small parallel echoes which pulsate. These parallel lines are in contact with the placenta at the cord insertion. Similarly, the fetal umbilicus can be visualized by condensation of these echoes next to the fetal abdomen. Information concerning the placental insertion of the cord is extremely helpful when one is choosing a site for amniocentesis in a patient with an anterior placenta.

Figure 11
Demonstration of umbilical vein.
Transverse section.

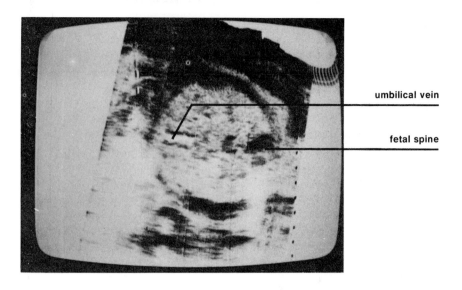

umbilical vein

fetal spine

Figure 12
Umbilical cord.

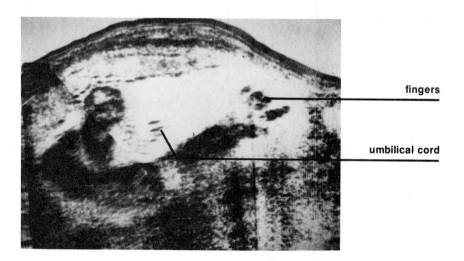

fingers

umbilical cord

The fetal heart is easily observed with real-time equipment, and M-mode studies of the fetal heart can be made using single transducers in the same way that they are made in the adult. With M-mode, it is not difficult to record sinusoid movements which arise from the annulus of the atrioventricular valves. The characteristic patterns of the atrioventricular and semi-lunar valves which are seen postnatally can frequently be identified. If one has identified the fetal spine and the fetal presentation, it is possible to distinguish the left side from the right side and, thus, distinguish the left ventricle from the right ventricle (Figure 13).

One may record characteristic echo patterns from the right ventricle, tricuspid valve, interventricular septum, mitral valve, and left ventricle simultaneously. Because of the variability of fetal position, the fortunate superimposition of these structures only occurs occasionally. However, the measurements obtained are of considerable theoretical interest, and this is a potentially useful way of measuring fetal cardiac output. Near term, in utero, the diameters of the left ventricular chamber can be measured, and these average about 13 mm. in diastole and 8 mm. in systole. After delivery, the diameter of the left ventricle increases substantially and measures about 18 mm. in diastole and 10 mm. in systole.

With simultaneous fetal electrocardiograms, it may be possible to measure the systolic time intervals in utero, in which case these may serve as indices of fetal well-being.

The heart serves as a good landmark for the thorax, and some investigators interested in measuring fetal body size have used a cross section at the level of the heart as an index of somatic growth. The heart, being on the left side, also serves as a landmark for the identification of the stomach (Figure 14), which can be seen as a transonic collection just beneath it.

Figure 13

Fetal echocardiogram.
Right ventricle, *rv*; left ventricle, *lv*; mitral valve, *m*; endocardium,
small arrows; epicardium, large arrows.

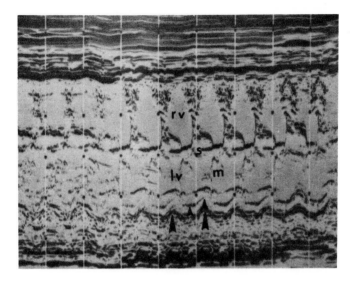

Figure 14

Fetal stomach.

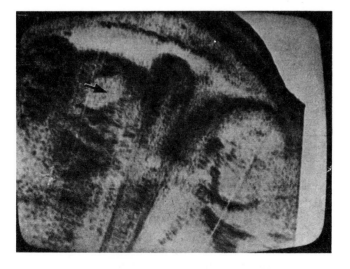

There is currently great interest in the study of fetal breathing. Investigators had first noticed thoracic excursions in the fetal lamb which seemed to correlate in pattern and frequency with fetal condition. Recently, some authors have reported their ability to demonstrate movements of the thoracic wall using A-mode. Three basic patterns are distinguished:

1   A normal pattern consists of somewhat irregular respirations of minimal amplitude occurring at a frequency of 40 to 70/min.
2   A mixed pattern consists of a combination of periods of the first pattern with periods of apnea. This has been associated with early fetal compromise.
3   An ominous pattern is described where there are large thoracic excursions, thought to represent gasping, which punctuate long periods of apnea.

These patterns have been correlated with fetal asphyxia. It is reported that respiratory movement diminishes when the patient smokes, that apnea also occurs prior to spontaneous labor, and that fetal respiratory movements are stimulated by glucose.

Although we have observed respiratory movements with real-time scanning and have recorded them cinegraphically, it is our impression that they are much less frequent than indicated in reports where A-mode is used (perhaps about 30% of the time). We have also observed that the respiratory movements are predominantly abdominal rather than thoracic, indicating mainly diaphragmatic movement. Hiccoughing is also seen from time to time and is not abnormal. It could well be confused with the so-called "gasping" pattern. As yet, there have been no systematic studies of respiratory movements using real-time equipment. These are needed since A-mode is an unreliable means of studying fetal respiration and prone to misinterpretation because of artifactual information.

When the position of the fetus is suitable, the fetal kidneys can be identified (Figure 15a). As in the adult, these kidneys contain a central acoustically reflecting mass produced by the calyceal-collecting systems and a relatively transonic cortex filled with urine. The kidneys are seen on each side of the acoustic shadow produced by the fetal spine.

Figure 15a
Normal fetal kidneys resembling "glasses over a nose."

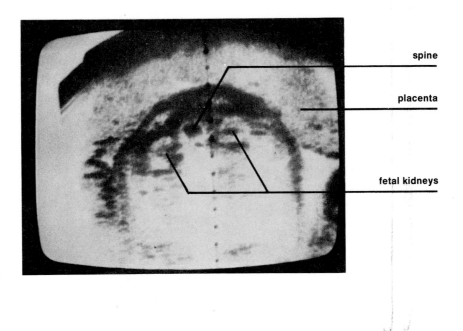

spine

placenta

fetal kidneys

Congenital cystic disease (Figure 15*b*) of the kidneys, as well as congenital hydronephrosis, are thus susceptible to ultrasonic diagnosis. The fetal bladder is an easy structure to identify when it is filled with urine (see Figure 4). With real-time scanning, the position of the fetal bladder and its volume are amenable to rapid measurement. As indicated in another chapter, serial measurements of bladder volume have been used to calculate the rate of urine production by Wladimiroff and Campbell. If there is renal agenesis, the bladder is not identified after repeated examination. In the presence of obstruction to the urethra, the urinary bladder is enlarged. It may also be enlarged in cases where the mother is receiving atropine-like medication.

A number of other congenital anomalies in utero have been reported, including abdominal cysts and intestinal obstruction. One would anticipate that with the accelerating use of ultrasound in obstetrics and the advances which are occurring in technology, the usefulness of ultrasound in diagnosis of congenital anomalies will increase (Figure 16).

Figure 15b

Abnormal fetal kidneys 3.5 MHz transducer. Transverse scan in
29-week fetus that was born with polycystic kidneys.

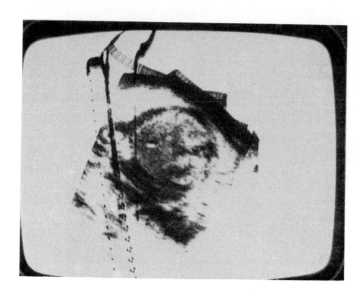

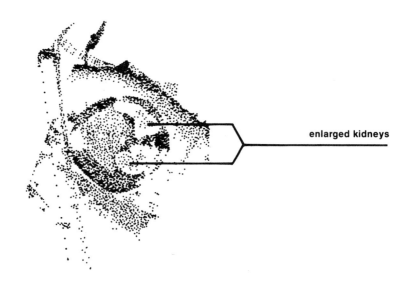

enlarged kidneys

Figure 16

A 28-week fetus with multiple anomalies.
Note massive fetal ascites.

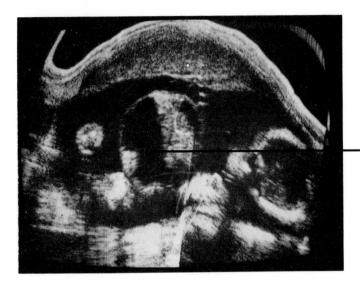

ascites

For the present, it is of considerable clinical importance to be able to diagnose urinary tract obstruction, renal agenesis, intestinal obstruction, hydrocephalus, anencephaly, and anomalies of the spinal column.

We should like to conclude this discussion of fetal anatomy and congenital anomalies with a note of caution. The medical, moral, and medico-legal consequences of making an ultrasonic diagnosis of congenital anomalies of the fetus are formidable. There have already been occasions (not reported in the literature) in which a false diagnosis of fetal anomaly has been made. Fluid-filled loops of bowel or stomach, for example, should not be called hydronephrotic kidneys. The ultrasonographer has to use his equipment responsibly, and, as his equipment improves, the community will expect a high level of competence.

Rh disease

Rh incompatibility is an important problem encountered in the second and third trimesters. Generally, ultrasonography is requested to find a site for amniocentesis, and here one wishes to avoid the placenta so as to prevent sensitization. However, when the placenta is anterior, it may be so bulky that no suitable site for amniocentesis can be found which does not require traversing the placenta. As the disease becomes more severe, the placenta becomes edematous and has a characteristic appearance in which the solid elements are separated by fluid spaces. As hydrops of the fetus develops, one sees a double outline of the fetal head produced by edema of the fetal scalp (Figure 17).

Late changes of erythroblastosis generally indicating irreversible disease include fetal ascites (Figure 18) and pericardial effusion. When there is fetal ascites, fluid is seen around the periphery of the abdomen displacing the abdominal organs medially. Pericardial effusion results in the finding of the heart surrounded by a halo of fluid. After intraperitoneal transfusion, an appearance similar to fetal ascites is observed due to the injection of blood into the peritoneal cavity. This regresses within a few days. The technique of intraperitoneal fetal transfusion using ultrasound is covered in another chapter.

Diabetes

Maternal diabetes constitutes a major threat to fetal survival, and the mechanism of death is still unknown. Patients who are glucose-intolerant only during pregnancy (gestational diabetics) and insulin-dependent diabetics without end-organ disease (nephropathy, retinopathy) tend to have large babies and large placentas. The current theory concerning the etiology of macrosomia is that the blood sugar in the fetus of the poorly controlled diabetic is periodically high, engendering excessive release of fetal insulin. This insulin stimulates fetal growth. Recent studies from Sweden indicate that fetal macrosomia can be obviated by scrupulous control of maternal blood sugars.

Ultrasound is an invaluable tool in monitoring the progress of these pregnancies, and fetal and placental findings correlate beautifully with biochemical tests of fetoplacental function such as urine estriol and serum HPL (human placental lactogen).

Figure 17
Hydropic fetus and placenta due to Rh disease.
Fetus died 5 days after this scan.

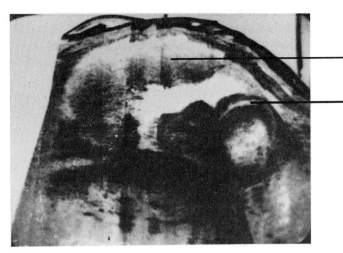

meaty edematous
placenta

double-
skull outline

Figure 18
Fetal ascites in Rh disease.
Transverse scan.

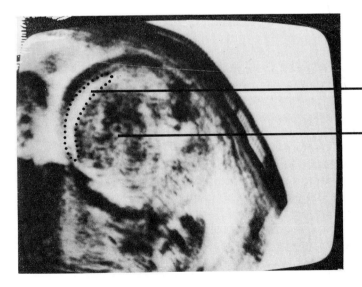

ascitic fluid

abdominal
contents

Total intrauterine volume in the macrosomic pregnancy is generally above the mean for gestation. With ultrasound, excess amniotic fluid is noted long before this can be appreciated clinically. If fluid accumulates rapidly, the placental volume will actually diminish, which is an ominous sign. Ultrasonic evidence of macrosomia indicates that the diabetic control is unsatisfactory.

The juvenile diabetic who has evidence of kidney or retinal disease often will deliver a small, withered baby and a sclerotic placenta. Intrauterine death occurs earlier in gestation in these patients than in the patient with less advanced disease whose macrosomic fetus rarely dies in utero before the 35th week of gestation. Although the patients with advanced diabetes frequently have high blood sugars, their babies will not become macrosomic because of concomitant placental insufficiency. Ultrasonic examination in these patients will reveal total intrauterine volumes to be either appropriate for dates or less than expected. Fetal dimensions may be small for dates, and the placental texture may be compatible with more advanced maturity. Often the fetus will be frankly growth-retarded, and in these cases tests of fetoplacental competence should be conducted as early as there is ultrasonic evidence of potential fetal compromise.

A subject which has received considerable attention in the literature is the effect of maternal diabetes on the biparietal diameters (BPD). There seems to be no unanimity of opinion as to whether biparietal diameters really are larger in macrosomic fetuses in late gestation. If BPDs are larger, is this a reflection of a large cranium, a thicker scalp, as suggested by Holländer, or both? It is our observation that BPDs are slightly larger in fetuses of diabetics, but this is rarely evidenced earlier than 34 weeks' gestation. This ultrasonic observation has been borne out by head circumference measurements at birth. Infants of diabetic mothers are large. They have large bones, large shoulders, and large pelvic dimensions. They also have excessive accumulation of adipose tissue in subcutaneous tissue and organomegaly. It would be safe to assume that the scalp thickness and the size of the calvarium both contribute to the larger biparietal diameters seen in macrosomic fetuses. The question could be easily put to rest if inner table measurements were compared in normal and diabetic pregnancies.

Certainly, we would suggest strongly that labor not be induced nor cesarean section be performed simply because the BPD is compatible with a mature fetus since BPDs are larger in diabetics, and fetuses of diabetic mothers tend to have delayed pulmonic maturity. In diabetes, the amniotic fluid L/S ratio is a preferable test of maturity. We have recently found that in 44% of diabetics where BPD was between 8.7 and 8.9 cm, the L/S ratio predicted pulmonic immaturity. Immature L/S ratios were found in 35% of patients where BPD was 9 or above.

Concomitant pelvic masses

Occasionally, pregnancy is complicated by a concomitant pelvic mass. Ultrasound is invaluable in evaluating the texture and size of these masses.

Ovarian cysts of all sizes can occur with pregnancy. In general, if the cyst is found in early pregnancy and is of sufficient size to warrant operation, it is judicious to postpone the procedure until the second trimester when the patient is less likely to abort. The reason for the lessened sensitivity of the uterus to manipulation after the 12th week is unknown. It originally was hypothesized that the ovary contributed progesterone to the maintenance of the early pregnancy, but subsequent studies of 17-hydroxyprogesterone, a product purely of ovarian origin, indicate that the ovary has little to do with gestational support after the 8th to 10th week. When an adnexal cyst is found in the second trimester, it is essential to measure its size. In general, if the cyst measures more than 6 cm. in any dimension, it is not going to regress during pregnancy, and exploratory laparotomy is indicated. If the cyst has solid components, operation should be undertaken. For example, on occasion we have been able to diagnose a cystic teratoma (dermoid) during pregnancy and have advised operation (Figure 19).

If the adnexal mass appears to be devoid of solid components and is less than 6 cm. in diameter, it is possible to follow the patient with serial scans through pregnancy. Often the cyst will diminish in size, obviating the need for exploratory laparotomy. Rupture of an ovarian cyst has been documented by ultrasound.

Figure 19
Dermoid cyst of ovary in cul-de-sac.

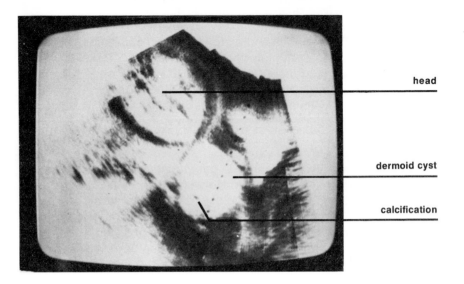

head

dermoid cyst

calcification

Sometimes a cyst will be noted for the first time in late pregnancy. If the cyst is thin-walled, one is concerned about rupture during labor, and, occasionally, it is large enough to obstruct the baby's descent. By scanning in many planes, it is possible to make a judgment on the probability of an obstructed labor, based on the size and location of the cyst.

With ultrasound evaluation, it is also possible to make the same assessment when pregnancy is complicated by other pelvic masses such as a pelvic kidney or a cervical fibroid. We recently had the opportunity to follow a pregnant patient with a renal transplant. The extra-peritoneally implanted kidney actually increased slightly in size during the later stage of gestation. Based on the experience of a few authors, we were prepared to deliver this patient vaginally. However, at about 38 weeks, ultrasonically-obtained information indicated that the baby could not progress through the pelvis unless there was significant compression of the transplanted kidney. The decision, therefore, was made to deliver this patient by cesarean section.

References

1 **Arger, P.H., and Zarembok, I.** Ultrasound efficacy in evaluation of lower genitourinary tract anomalies. J. Clin. Ultrasound 3:61, 1975.

2 **Barker, P., and Cashman, D.** Diagnosis of multiple pregnancy. Br. Med. J. 2:487, 1973.

3 **Burton, B.K., Gerbie, A.B., and Nadler, H.L.** Present status of intrauterine diagnosis of genetic defects. Am. J. Obstet. Gynecol. 118:718, 1974.

4 **Campbell, S., Johnstone, F.D., Holt, E.M., and May, P.** Anencephaly: early ultrasonic diagnosis and active management. Lancet 2:1226, 1972.

5 **Campbell, S., Wladimiroff, J.W., and Dewhurst, C.J.** The antenatal measurement of fetal urine production. J. Obstet. Gynaecol. Br. Commonw. 80:680, 1973.

6 **Dawes, G.S.** Breathing before birth in animals and man. An essay in developmental medicine. N. Engl. J. Med. 290:557, 1974.

7 **Editorial:** Antenatal diagnosis of spina bifida. Br. Med. J. 1:414, 1975.

8 **Farman, K.J., and Thomas, G.** The use of ultrasound for monitoring foetal breathing movements. Biomed. Eng. (N.Y.) 10:172, 1975.

9 **Field, B., Mitchell, G., Garrett, W., and Kerr, C.** Letter: amniotic alpha-fetoprotein levels and anencephaly. Lancet 2:798, 1973.

10 **Garrett, W.J., Grunwald, G., and Robinson, D.E.** Prenatal diagnosis of fetal polycystic kidney by ultrasound. Aust. N.Z. J. Obstet. Gynaecol. 10:7, 1970.

11 **Garrett, W.J., Kossoff, G., and Osborn, R.A.** The diagnosis of fetal hydronephrosis, megaureter and urethral obstruction by ultrasonic echography. Br. J. Obstet. Gynaecol. 82:115, 1975.

12 **Garrett, W.J., and Robinson, D.E.** Fetal heart size measured in vivo by ultrasound. Pediatrics 46:25, 1970.

13 **Gottesfeld, K.R.** The ultrasonic diagnosis of intrauterine fetal death. Am. J. Obstet. Gynecol. 108:623, 1970.

14 **Holländer.** Ultrasound in the prenatal diagnosis of Rh erythroblastosis. World Congress of Ultrasound in Medicine, Vienna, 1969.

15 **Hon, E.H., Murata, Y., Zanini, B., Martin, C.B., Jr., and Lewis, D.E.** Continuous microfilm display of the electromechanical intervals of the cardiac cycle. Obstet. Gynecol. 43:722, 1974.

16 **Jouppila, P., Ylostalo, P., and Pystynen, P.** Fetal head growth measured by ultrasound in the last few weeks of pregnancy in normal, toxaemic and diabetic women. Acta Obstet. Gynecol. Scand. 49:367, 1970.

17 **Kossoff, G., and Garrett, W.J.** Intracranial detail in fetal echograms. Invest. Radiol. 7:159, 1972.

18 **Kratochwil, A., and Schaller, A.** Obstetric diagnostics of anencephalus using ultrasound. Geburtshilfe Frauenheilkd. 31:564, 1971.

19 **Kratochwil, A., Stroger, H., and Schaller, A.** Obstetrical ultrasonic diagnosis of hydrocephalus. Geburtshilfe Frauenheilkd. 33:322, 1973.

20 **Laurence, K.M.** Fetal malformations and abnormalities. Lancet 2:939, 1974.

21 **Lorber, J., Stewart, C.R., and Ward, A.M.** Alpha-fetoprotein in antenatal diagnosis of anencephaly and spina bifida. Lancet 1:1187, 1973.

22 **Michell, R.C., and Bradley-Watson, P.J.** The detection of fetal meningocoele by ultrasound B scan. J. Obstet. Gynaecol. Br. Commonw. 80:1100, 1973.

23 **Murata, Y., and Martin, C.B., Jr.** Systolic time intervals of the fetal cardiac cycle. Obstet. Gynecol. 44:224, 1974.

24 **Organ, L.W., Bernstein, A., Smith, K.C., and Rowe, I.H.** The preejection period of the fetal heart: patterns of change during labor. Am. J. Obstet. Gynecol. 120:49, 1974.

25 **Papp, Z., Berta, I., and Arvay, A.** Early antenatal diagnosis of anencephaly. Lancet 1:729, 1973.

26 **Winsberg, F.** Echocardiography of the fetal and newborn heart. Invest. Radiol. 7:152, 1972.

Abnormal Growth and Development

6

Today it is possible not only to diminish perinatal mortality, but to improve the quality of life of our offspring. Intrauterine growth retardation (IUGR) represents a significant threat to that quality of life. IUGR complicates 3 to 7% of all pregnancies in the United States and Canada. Higher incidences are reported in predominantly indigent populations with poor nutrition, in heavy smokers, and where pregnancy occurs in the presence of drug addiction or alcoholism. No socioeconomic class, however, is excluded when pregnancy is accompanied by chronic hypertension, advanced diabetes, toxemia, or the rarely encountered entity, primary placental disease.

A baby is considered growth-retarded when it is in or below the 10th percentile of mean weight for gestation at birth. These babies have an eight-fold increase in perinatal mortality and a four-fold increase in intrapartum asphyxia, and present the pediatrician with significant neonatal problems of acidosis, hypoglycemia, hypocalcemia, and polycythemia. It is of great concern that many of these babies will also have neurological sequelae which emerge in infancy and childhood. In order to change the course of IUGR, the condition must be diagnosed early in pregnancy rather than at birth.

Babies are growth-retarded for one of three basic reasons:

1 The mother is nutritionally deficient.
2 Maternal nutrition is adequate, but the placenta is incapable of transferring nutrient to the fetus. This occurs in such conditions complicating pregnancy as toxemia, chronic hypertension, severe diabetes, and renal disease.
3 The baby is genetically deformed or has been subjected at an early stage of development to an intrauterine insult such as viral infection, drugs, or other biochemical agents. This accounts for 10% of all cases of IUGR.

In rats, one can experimentally produce two different types of IUGR, reflected by head and body configuration, by manipulating maternal nutrition or blood flow to the uterus. The rat born to the nutritionally deficient mother is symmetrically small, and brain cell number, as determined by DNA content, is significantly diminished. The rats born after diminishing uterine blood flow are asymmetrically small. The trunk and internal organs are significantly depleted of DNA when compared with the brain, which is relatively spared.

Recently, Stuart Campbell, a significant contributor in the field of obstetrical ultrasonics, described two types of abnormal growth patterns in humans which are remarkably similar to those produced in rats. In one pattern, exhibited in 20 to 30% of small-for-dates babies, there was a lag in both biparietal diameter (BPD) and trunk area throughout the third trimester ("low profile growth"). In the other pattern, biparietal diameter was only diminished very late in the gestation, thus creating a picture of disproportion between head and body. The asymmetrical fetuses were more prone to perinatal asphyxia, while the symmetrical fetuses behaved no differently in labor than normal fetuses. Occasionally, the very small fetuses were anomalous.

Our observations

1   In an ongoing study to monitor pregnancies at risk for IUGR with ultrasound, it has been our distinct impression that in most cases, regardless of the cause, the fetus will first spare its brain at the expense of its body. In other words, whether the problem is malnutrition in a patient with pernicious vomiting, or placental perfusion is compromised as a result of hypertension, the first ultrasonic sign of compromise is disproportion between head and body (Figure 1). If the pathological process is allowed to continue, the fetus will be unable to compensate by sparing its brain, and *then* there will be a lag in cranial growth. There may be a critical threshold for each patient involving the type of insult, the duration of the insult, and the tolerance of the fetus. When this threshold is exceeded, the brain is no longer spared. The exception to this rule is the congenitally deformed fetus, who frequently will demonstrate the earliest evidence of symmetrical growth lag or an occasional baby that is genetically small. However, with the exclusion of anomalous fetuses, it is rare for a significant biparietal diameter lag to occur prior to the 30th week of gestation except in severe intrauterine

Figure 1

Fetus with severe intrauterine growth retardation.
Note disproportion between head and body.

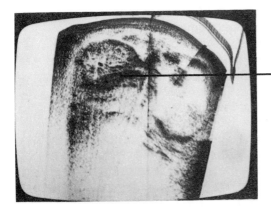

spine

deprivation. In these cases of severe IUGR it is
unusual for perinatal asphyxia *not* to occur.

2 Retarded growth is often accompanied by other
ultrasonic findings, such as diminished amniotic fluid
resulting in fetal crowding. This is appreciated by a
diminished distance between crown and rump and
the separation of fetal small parts by very small
amounts of amniotic fluid. With real-time scanning,
one can note a diminished amplitude of fetal limb
motion. These findings most often precede
diminution of biparietal diameter growth by many
weeks (except when the pregnancy is complicated by
diabetes) and can often be appreciated only by the
experienced observer.

3 Measurements of the abdominal girth are extremely
useful in assessing the degree of compromise in the
fetus, and this measurement correlates well with fetal
weight (see Appendix).

4 In 50% of cases of IUGR, the placenta is smaller than
expected for its stage of gestation, and this visual
impression can be quantitatively assessed by
measurements of placental volume described below.
Also, the placental texture in these compromised
pregnancies is compatible with a more mature
pregnancy.

5 We have found the determination of total intrauterine
volume (TIUV), which reflects any or all of the above
changes, to be an invaluable predictor of IUGR. This
will be described later in the chapter.

Ultrasonic dimensions
Fetus
Serial BPD determinations Although it is essential to perform these measurements every 2 to 3 weeks when IUGR is suspected, the usefulness of these examinations is enhanced immeasurably when utilized in combination with the other measurements described below.

Let us discuss some of the pitfalls of measuring BPD alone. Since BPD growth often is affected last in the sequence of diagnostic clues associated with IUGR, the fetus already may be severely compromised when a lag in BPD is demonstrated. Because of the phenomenon of brain sparing, the incidence of false negatives is 21% when plateauing BPDs are used as the only criterium of IUGR. On the other hand, it is surprising, at first glance, that Campbell reports an 18% incidence of false positives when the BPD growth is below the 10th percentile in the last 10 weeks of pregnancy. However, let us remember that BPD growth normally tapers off in the last month of pregnancy to a mean of 1.3 mm./week and that the standard error of the method (about $\pm$ 2 mm.) at this time precludes one's ability to make a statistical judgment based on two BPD measurements less than 3 weeks apart in late gestation.

It is a distinct advantage to have a BPD measurement when there are early clinical signs of IUGR because it can be used to validate dates and to establish a baseline for serial studies. When comparing head to body ratios, it is more appropriate to use circumference or area measurements of the head (see Appendix).

Thorax Some investigators have used this measurement to predict fetal age and/or weight (see Appendix). The advantages of this method are that the chest is not easily compressed, and one can identify the proper plane to measure by using the fetal heart as a reference point (Figures 2a and 2b). However, the tissue densities within the thorax are so heterogeneous and the outline so irregular that it is often difficult to identify precisely outer boundaries. This cross-sectional measurement is useful but offers fewer discrete endpoints than circumference or area measurements of the abdomen.

Figure 2a

Sagittal scan demonstrating planes for transverse scanning to obtain thoracic and abdominal circumference measurements.

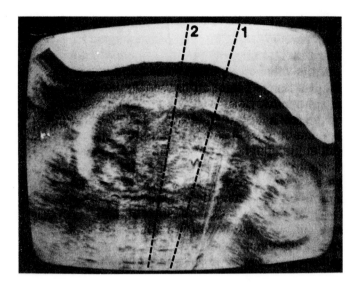

Figure 2b

Thoracic circumference when transverse scan performed at level 1.

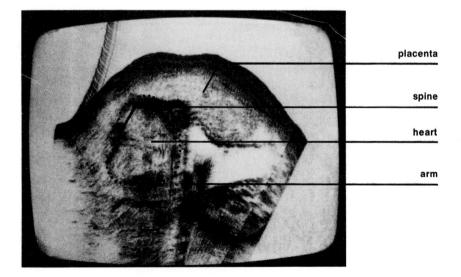

placenta

spine

heart

arm

Figure 2c

Abdominal circumference at level of umbilical vein scanned at level 2.

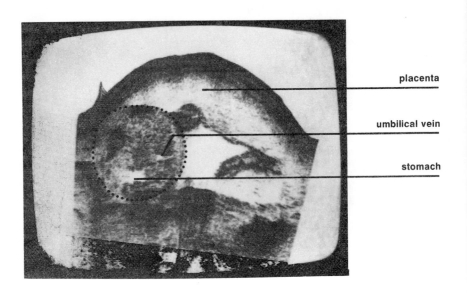

placenta

umbilical vein

stomach

Abdomen With gray scale and real-time the umbilical vein can be consistently recognized when scanning at right angles to the fetal spine, and measurements of area or circumference can be made at this level (Figures 2a and 2c). Generally, the liver can be seen in this plane, but its outline is difficult to delineate. With more sophisticated instrumentation, however, it may be possible to measure fetal liver area. This measurement would be particularly valuable since a growth-retarded baby will deprive its liver before other parts of the body or organs are affected by lack of proper nutrient.

In IUGR, cross-sectional body areas are generally diminished in comparison with biparietal diameters or head circumference measurements. A ratio of head circumference to body circumference is of definite value. This ratio normally changes as pregnancy progresses. In the second trimester, the head circumference is larger than that of the abdomen, but at about 32 to 36 weeks the ratio equals unity, and the body measurement becomes proportionately larger after 36 weeks. It must be remembered that if scans are not made exactly at right angles to the sagittal line of the fetus, it is possible to affect the measurements by these tangential cuts. As reported by Campbell, we have found that up until the 37th week of gestation, the abdominal circumference correlates extremely well with fetal weight (see Appendix).

Total intrauterine volume (TIUV)

Some time ago, it occurred to us that even though the intrauterine contents are not affected by intrauterine deprivation in a parallel fashion, a diminution of incremental growth of each or all would be represented in their sum, the TIUV. It is quite possible to measure this volume with a three-dimensional formula for volume of an ellipse. One simply scans across the abdomen sagittally until the largest diameter between anterior and posterior uterine walls is found. In this plane, this dimension and the distance between the top of the fundus and a point at the level of the internal cervical os are recorded (Figure 3a). A transverse measurement is made between the uterine side walls (Figure 3b), and the volume is computed from these three dimensions by the formula:

$$V = 4/3\,\pi \left(\frac{\text{Diameter A}}{2} \times \frac{B}{2} \times \frac{C}{2} \right)$$

condensed to $V = 0.523 \times ABC$.

Since the dimensional endpoints are somewhat inexact, it must be remembered that this volume determination is not extremely precise. It, however, is accurate enough to obtain very useful information. To test the method, we have measured the amount of amniotic fluid drained by amniocentesis in patients with polyhydramnios and found that the difference between determinations of TIUV before and after the amniocentesis was within 75 cc. of the amount of fluid withdrawn.

TIUV increases in normal pregnancy as indicated in the Appendix. It is of note that TIUV rapidly increases near term at a time when BPD growth normally has tapered off. We have found that the earliest sign of IUGR is the lack of expected increase in TIUV, which is generally a result of growth lag of the fetal trunk and diminution of amniotic fluid volume. Thus far, if the TIUV lags behind the BPD by 4 weeks or more, all of these babies have been growth-retarded at birth (Figure 4). That is to say, if TIUV is below 1 1/2 standard deviations below dates (validated by BPD), the fetus is

Figure 3a
Dimensions for measurement of TIUV.
Sagittal scan.

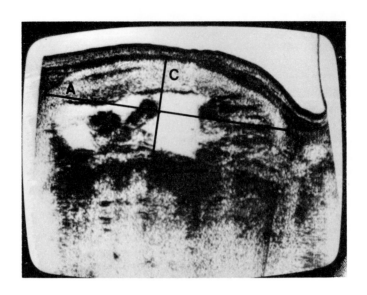

Figure 3b
Dimensions for measurement of TIUV.
Transverse scan.

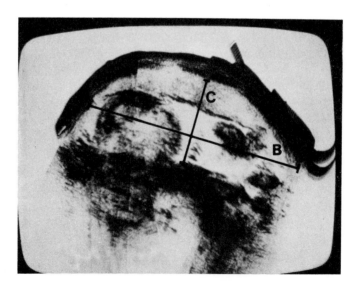

growth-retarded. In symmetrical IUGR, the ratio between BPD and TIUV is less divergent, but the BPD then lags behind the patient's dates. The placenta, if small, may also contribute to the disparity between TIUV and dates. With TIUV and BPD alone, most cases of IUGR can be diagnosed.

Figure 4

Total intrauterine volume.

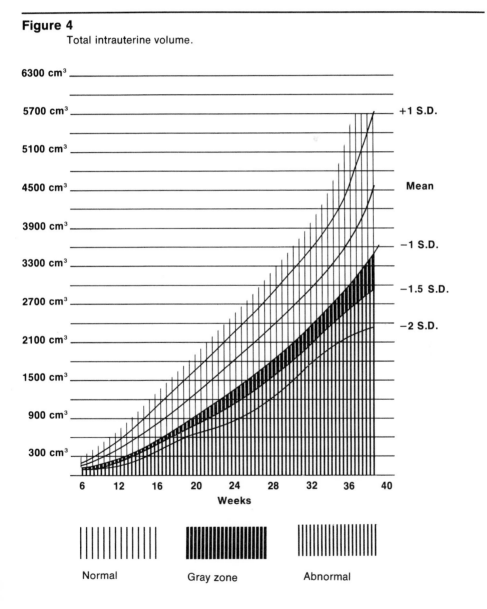

Normal   Gray zone   Abnormal

Placenta

In about 50% of cases of IUGR, the placenta is small. As mentioned earlier, the texture of the growth-retarded placenta is different from that of the normal placenta at the same stage of gestation. With higher frequency transducers (3.5 MHz and 5 MHz), it is now possible to delineate the architecture of anterior and fundal placentas and to develop a pathological scoring system or maturity index based on placental texture and architecture. Infarctions or calcifications and signs of abruption can also be appreciated.

Growth of the normal placenta can be traced ultrasonically. To measure placental growth, one scans sagittally across the abdomen until the longest diameter of the placenta is found (Figure 5a). The placenta is also generally thickest in this plane since the placenta has the configuration of a pancake (planoconvex). A transverse scan is performed at right angles to the above plane at the point where the placenta was noted to be the thickest by sagittal scan (Figure 5b). The width of the placenta is then recorded. Each measurement may be plotted serially and placental volume determined from the above measurements by the following formula:
$V = \pi/6 \, C \, (3/4 \, AB + C^2)$. Anterior placentas are the easiest to measure. Fundal and posterior placentas present a problem and often require semi-quantitative estimation of dimensions. A nomogram for placental volume has been constructed by Hellman and Kobayashi and is presented in the Appendix.

We have found measurement of the individual placental dimensions to be of value. In normal pregnancies, the placental length and width increase linearly throughout gestation. Although placental thickness varies from patient to patient, the dimension of thickness increases linearly until about the 34th to 37th week of gestation, and then it actually diminishes. For example, the placenta may attain a thickness of 4.5 cm. in late pregnancy and then shrink to about 3.5 cm. One may speculate as to why this interesting phenomenon occurs. It has been demonstrated that about the same time the placenta is at its thickest, there is no further cell multiplication. Hypertrophy of each placental cell continues, however. Therefore, it seems that the placenta spreads itself out, perhaps in a compensatory effort to be in contact with more surface. It does this at the expense of its thickness. In abnormal pregnancies such as toxemia, entirely different growth patterns are often noted, depending upon the severity of the

Figure 5a

Dimensions for measurement of placental volume.
Sagittal scan.
Note thin placenta.

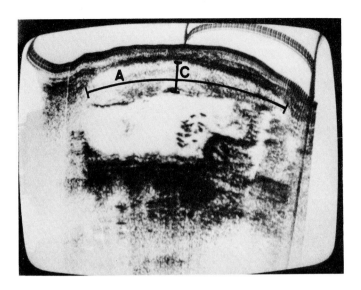

Figure 5b

Dimensions for measurement of placental volume.
Transverse scan.

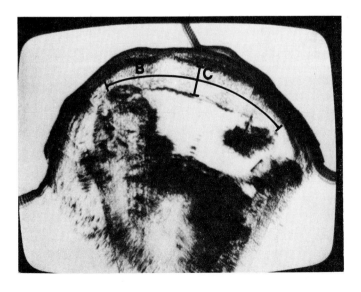

condition. In placental compromise, the dimensions of length and width will generally stabilize, and the placenta will not become thinner. In some cases, there will be no further growth of the placenta at all, and 2 weeks later the volume will be the same. These plotted ultrasonic changes promise to provide the physician with more information concerning the condition of the placenta in jeopardized pregnancies and can be correlated with biochemical indices of placental function.

Fetal urine production

Campbell initially reported a method to quantitate fetal urine production using three-dimensional determinations of bladder volume (Figures 6a and 6b). The formula for bladder volume is identical to that described for TIUV. He found that it was possible, with two measurements obtained at 20- to 30-min. intervals, to compute urine accumulation in the bladder per hour, termed hourly fetal urinary production rate (HFUPR). After establishing a normal curve for different times of gestation (Appendix), he was able, in a subsequent paper, to correlate diminished HFUPR with IUGR. There are some distinct difficulties encountered in determining HFUPR. First of all, although the method appears to be simple to perform, it is time-consuming and must be performed precisely. When the bladder outline is clearly discerned sagittally, the patient's abdomen is marked and the angle noted over the deepest dimension of the bladder. When the ultrasonographer scans transversely in this plane, the measurement of the depth may be smaller than the sagittal depth dimension. At first, we felt this simply was a result of poor technique, but, subsequently, through the revelation of real-time ultrasound, we realized that the fetus and its bladder move during the examination. We now use real-time exclusively for this determination because it is not only faster, but more precise, since one determination often would take 10 min. to perform with compound contact scanning, and bladder volume changes during this period of time.

The reader should also keep in mind that in order to perform HFUPR measurements the patient is often on her back for prolonged periods of time, and uterine blood flow is diminished. Therefore, the scan should be performed as expeditiously as possible, and the patient should be allowed to lie on her side between scans.

This is not an examination that has clinical efficacy in a large percentage of patients, and, at present, we

Figure 6a

Dimensions for measurement of bladder volume.

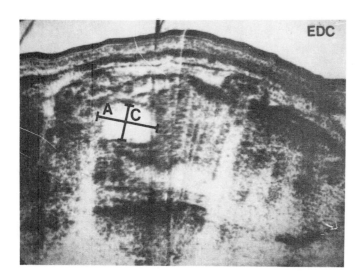

Figure 6b

Transverse scan of bladder.

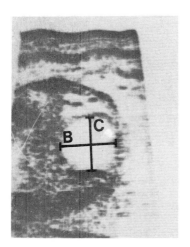

Scheme for evaluation of a patient at risk for IUGR

Initial Examination TIUV and BPD	Fetal Dimensions	Serial Examination	Diagnosis	Disposition
1. Dates, BPD, TIUV all within 2 weeks of each other			No IUGR	Discharge
2. BPD and dates greater than TIUV by 1½ to 3 weeks		Appropriate growth of BPD and TIUV	No IUGR	Discharge
		TIUV now lags BPD by 4 weeks or more	Early IUGR	Go to Growth Profile 4
3. Dates greater than BPD by 3 weeks or more; BPD and TIUV within 2 weeks of each other		Appropriate growth of BPD and TIUV	Incorrect dates No IUGR	Due date changed
		Inappropriate growth of both BPD and TIUV	Correct dates Severe IUGR	Go to Growth Profile 5
4. BPD and dates greater than TIUV by 4 weeks or more	Head-to-body disproportion	No lag of BPD	Early IUGR	Weekly OCTs; Biochemical monitoring; Weekly L/S ratios when feasible
		BPD now lags dates by more than 2 weeks	Severe IUGR	Bed rest in lateral recumbent position
5. Dates greater than BPD by more than 2 weeks; BPD greater than TIUV by more than 3 weeks	All dimensions small	No further lag in BPD	Severe IUGR	
		Further lag in BPD	Severe IUGR (look for anomalies)	
	Head-to-body disproportion	Lag in BPD	Severe IUGR	
		No lag in BPD	Incorrect dates with early IUGR	

have used the technique exclusively as a research tool. HFUPR seems to correlate best with body size, which, in turn, may be predicted best by measurements of abdominal girth.

Scheme for IUGR

The following is a somewhat detailed discussion of the diagnostic regimen outlined for the reader's reference. The numbered statements apply to the numbers in the outline. The patients at risk for IUGR are first referred for a routine diagnostic scan and determination of TIUV, when utilized. A full growth profile consists of circumference measurements of head, thorax, abdominal circumference, placental volume, and, occasionally, HFUPR.

1   Sixty per cent of patients have normal TIUVs and BPDs appropriate for dates, even when the uterus appears clinically to be smaller than dates. Often the baby is in an oblique or transverse lie, which tends to affect the clinical measurement between the symphysis and fundus. Occasionally, the uterus seems small because the fetus' head has dipped into the pelvis. No further scans are necessary if the TIUV and BPD concur with the patient's dates.

2   Often the TIUV lags behind the patient's dates (and BPD) by 1 1/2 to 3 weeks. This is within the observed variation of normal. The patient should have another routine exam and TIUV in 2 weeks. If the baby is growth-retarded, the discrepancy between TIUV and dates (BPD) will then be more than 3 weeks. Fortunately, in most cases, on repeat exam the TIUV is within 2 weeks of the BPD, and IUGR is excluded.

3   If TIUV lags BPD by less than 2 weeks, but there is a disparity between the patient's dates and BPD by more than 3 weeks, it is likely that the patient's dates are incorrect. Another examination is performed in 2 to 3 weeks, and if there is appropriate growth of both TIUV and BPD over that period of time, the patient's due date is changed. If parallel inappropriate growth of both BPD and TIUV is encountered during the interval, then the fetus has severe symmetrical growth retardation; and the patient is scheduled for a full growth profile. These fetuses should be delivered when there is reasonable chance of extrauterine survival.

4   If TIUV lags behind BPD by more than 3 weeks, then a growth profile is performed; and the patient is committed to ultrasonic examinations every 2 to 3

weeks until delivery. She is encouraged to spend much of her day in the lateral recumbent position. The majority of these babies will have head-to-body disproportion, and 50%°will have small placentas. On repeat exam, some of the borderline cases (TIUV initially lagged BPD by 3 to 4 weeks) will now fall within the normal range. In these cases, one more exam is required in 3 weeks. Most cases, however, continue to exhibit a disparity; and, often, in severe disease, the BPD begins to lag behind the patient's dates.

5   If BPD lags behind dates by more than 2 weeks, and there is more than 3 weeks disparity between BPD and TIUV, one is often dealing with a severe form of growth retardation. Occasionally, however, this combination of factors is noted in early IUGR in a patient who is also mistaken on her dates. A full growth profile is performed, and the extent of intrauterine deprivation can be assessed by a determination of abdominal circumference and head-to-body ratio.

In cases where there is symmetrically retarded fetal growth, it is important to look for congenital anomalies, as there are current methods such as amniography and amniotic fluid alpha-fetoprotein determinations which can identify some types of congenital anomalies. A scan of the spine should be accomplished to look for large spinal defects. It is particularly useful in cases where scant amounts of amniotic fluid are found to perform HFUPR. If there is renal agenesis or non-functioning polycystic kidneys, a fetal bladder will not be noted. It should be pointed out, however, that one should scan the patient at 15-min. intervals for more than $1\frac{1}{2}$ hr. before the diagnosis of non-functioning kidneys can be made.

With the oxytocin challenge test, one can determine the status of the fetoplacental unit by initiating contractions in the patient with pitocin. If the fetal heart rate does not drop after a contraction, this has been a reliable indicator that in utero demise will not occur within 1 week of the test. If contractions do produce this characteristic pattern in fetal heart rate (positive OCT), the fetus could be in severe jeopardy. Although the incidence of false positives (positive OCT's in patients whose babies had no evidence of distress during labor) has been reported to be as high as 50%, it is best to deliver the baby with IUGR if the OCT is positive.

In our experience, it is possible, in some cases, to improve fetal growth in utero by improving maternal nutrition, treating some of the conditions responsible for the IUGR, and by improving uterine blood flow by liberal prescriptions for rest in a lateral recumbent position. We have recently demonstrated on ten occasions a salutary effect on TIUV by bed rest in this position.

Each case, however, should be considered separately, and the decision to deliver should be based on the severity of IUGR, the pulmonary status of the fetus (L/S ratio to be discussed in a subsequent chapter), and the results of biochemical indices of fetoplacental well-being. In most cases of IUGR, especially where there is evidence of fetal pulmonic maturity, it would be more judicious to deliver the patient and allow the baby to be fed in a newborn special care unit than to subject it to any further time in an alien intrauterine environment.

References

1 **Campbell, S.** Fetal urine production. J. Obstet. Gynaecol. Br. Commonw. 80:680, 1973.

2 **Campbell, S.** Physical methods of assessing size at birth. In *Size at Birth,* Ciba Foundation Symposium 27. Associated Scientific Publishers, Amsterdam, 1974.

3 **Campbell, S., and Dewhurst, C.J.** Diagnosis of the small-for-dates fetus by serial ultrasonic cephalometry. Lancet 2:1002, 1971.

4 **Gohari, P., Berkowitz, R.L., and Hobbins, J.C.** Prediction of intrauterine growth retardation by determination of total intrauterine volume. Am. J. Obstet. Gynecol. 127:255, 1977.

5 **Levi, S., and Erbsman, F.** Antenatal fetal growth from the nineteenth week. Ultrasonic study of 12 head and chest dimensions. Am. J. Obstet. Gynecol. 121:262, 1975.

6 **Levi, S., and Smets, P.** Intrauterine fetal growth studied by ultrasonic biparietal measurements. Acta Obstet. Gynecol. Scand. 52:193, 1973.

7 **Winnick, M., and Noble P.** Quantitative changes in DNA and RNA and protein during prenatal and postnatal growth in the rat. Dev. Biol. 12:451, 1965.

Amniocentesis

7

Ultrasound plays an essential role in many special obstetrical techniques. This chapter deals with methods used to assess the condition and maturity of the fetus and to treat it should these tests indicate fetal jeopardy.

At first glance, some of the material included in this chapter may seem inappropriate in a text on ultrasound. Nonetheless, we feel that care of the patient should not be fragmented, and the technician or physician who plays an essential role in obtaining amniotic fluid should certainly have a basic knowledge of why the tap is being performed.

Our knowledge of the fetus has increased appreciably over the past few years, and probably the greatest reason for this recent insight into fetal status has been the availability of amniotic fluid. The fetus is protected by it, excretes and sheds cells into it, breathes it, swallows it, and may even obtain nourishment from it. Despite the recent inroads in obtaining fetal information from specific constituents of amniotic fluid, the dynamics of this mystery fluid are still poorly understood. For instance, we know that the fetus at term will swallow about 450 cc./day, but it may swallow greater amounts if there is a large amniotic fluid volume or if there is uterine irritability. This, however, is obviously not the only pathway of removal. It has been demonstrated that the half-life of water in amniotic fluid is 95 min., indicating an aqueous turnover of 480 ml./hr. or approximately 11,000 cc./day. Therefore, at most, fetal swallowing accounts for 1/20th of the total turnover of water in the amniotic fluid. The fetal membranes undoubtedly are quite permeable to certain amniotic fluid components, and one group of investigators has even recently reported transfer of amino acids across the umbilical cord, indicating that extra fetal transfer of amniotic fluid constituents is not just reserved for substances of low molecular weight.

Certainly, not all is known about the mechanisms of amniotic fluid formation. There is no doubt, for instance, that the kidney contributes to the contents and volume of amniotic fluid; and, as stated earlier, it has recently been demonstrated by ultrasonic studies that the human fetus at term normally micturates more than 28 cc./hr. into the amniotic fluid. The fetal lung may even play some part in the formation of amniotic fluid. Animal studies, in fact, have demonstrated that the fetal lamb can secrete copious quantities of tracheal fluid. Yet these two contributors cannot account for the volume changes and exchange rates of individual components of amniotic fluid, and perhaps more precise knowledge of the origin and destination of specific amniotic fluid components will enable us to learn even more about the fetus.

Second trimester amniocentesis

Amniocentesis can be performed as early as the 14th week of gestation if the uterine fundus has risen above the symphysis pubis. It was initially assumed in prenatal genetic evaluation that the earlier the amniocentesis the better, since a karyotype could not be performed until after 14 to 24 days of cell culture growth. If the cells failed to grow, the amniocentesis would have to be repeated, followed by the same delay until karyotyping could be accomplished. In most cytogenetic tissue culture labs, however, it is rare for culture failures to occur; and if the cells are not thriving, this can be recognized within a few days of the tap. The procedure is also safer when it is postponed until about the 16th week of gestation, because there is more amniotic fluid (about 175 cc.) at this time, and there are more options for tapping sites. After this time, one must consider the psychological disadvantages to the patient.

We have found ultrasonic localization of a suitable area for amniocentesis to be essential in the second trimester tap. A pocket of amniotic fluid away from the fetal vital parts and placenta can generally be found with ease. In about 40% of cases, the placenta is implanted anteriorly. However, because the placenta may not cover the entire anterior surface of the uterus, it is possible to find a placenta-free area to penetrate in about half of these cases. When placental penetration is unavoidable, it is preferable to choose a peripheral extension of the placenta to traverse (Figure 1). Here, there is little risk of penetrating the umbilical cord where it inserts on the placenta or the large fetal vessels in the adjacent area of the chorionic plate. With gray scale or real-time imaging, one can often locate the placental insertion of the cord (Figure 2).

Figure 1

Sagittal scan of 16-week gestation.
Selected needle pathway represented by gradicule.

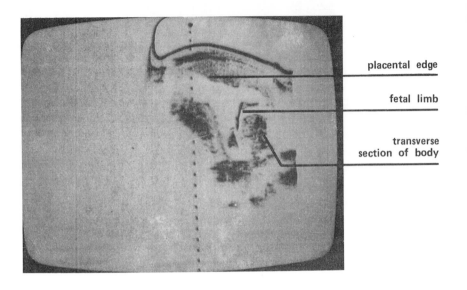

placental edge

fetal limb

transverse
section of body

Figure 2

Anterior placenta in 15-week pregnancy.
Note central insertion of umbilical cord.

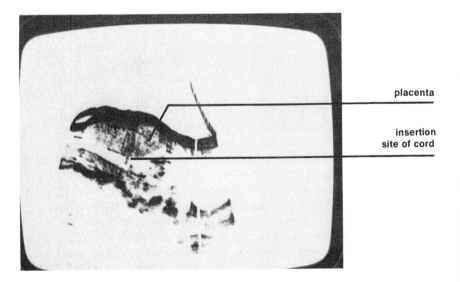

placenta

insertion
site of cord

Pockets of amniotic fluid depend upon the position of the fetus, and often it is advantageous to move the fetus to create another pocket of fluid in a more desirable location. Occasionally, the fetal head occupies an area under a placenta-free window. In these cases, one can maneuver the fetus into another position and perform the tap rapidly before the fetus moves back into the vacated space.

The dilated uterine vessels are to be avoided; therefore, in the second trimester tap, we strongly suggest that the operator not stray too far from either side of the midline. In fact, it is preferable to penetrate the placenta rather than tap too far laterally. It is extremely useful for the patient to have a full bladder because it facilitates visualization of the intrauterine contents and elevates the uterus out of the pelvis.

Method

The needle insertion site is marked on the patient's abdomen. The distance between the anterior abdominal wall and a point in the middle of the amniotic fluid pocket is recorded, and the angle of insertion is noted (Figure 3). We find it essential to display the appropriate scan on the television screen for reference. Logically, the larger the needle diameter the greater the potential trauma; therefore, it is preferable to use a 20- or 22-gauge needle. Most disposable spinal needles are 9 cm. from hub to tip. In the very obese patient, a longer needle is required.

Since one of the greatest contributors to morbidity is sepsis, it is imperative to maintain scrupulously aseptic technique. For instance, mineral oil should not be used prior to a tap unless it is removed with acetone. After the abdomen is prepared with an antiseptic solution and the skin is infiltrated with a local anesthetic (with a 22-gauge needle, local anesthesia is not necessary, and one of the authors [F.W.] no longer employs it), the needle is inserted into the uterine cavity. The operator should feel each tissue layer as it is being penetrated. We have found it necessary to advance the needle about 1 cm. more than the previously measured distance. This is difficult to explain, but there are three possible reasons:

1   There is some compression of the skin by the transducer during the scan.
2   The skin tents up along the needle as it is inserted.
3   The local anesthesia increases the thickness of the tissue.

Figure 3

Posterior placenta.
Selected pathway of needle represented by gradicule.
Ideal distance to center of fluid pocket, 6 cm.

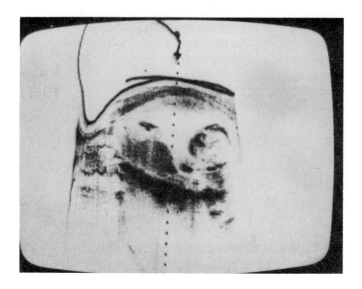

In any case, the stylet should be removed only when the desired distance is attained; then, if the cavity has been entered cleanly, clear fluid will appear at the needle hub.

Blood may interfere with cell growth in the mid-trimester amniocentesis. If the first syringe contains bloody fluid, another sample of fluid should be withdrawn into another syringe. If bloody fluid is still obtained, syringes should be changed until clear fluid is obtained. Even in the 20% of cases where an anterior placenta is penetrated, it is rare not to obtain clear fluid with the above technique, since the blood clots rapidly on the placental surface. We suggest that the syringe be disengaged before the needle is removed from the abdomen, since blood can be inadvertently drawn into the syringe as the needle is pulled back.

With the above technique, performed in the ultrasound laboratory, we have diminished appreciably our incidence of bloody taps (a bloody tap is defined as any visible blood in the amniotic fluid) and our number of needle insertions per patient. Morbidity increases with the number of unsuccessful amniocentesis attempts.

In bloody taps, the fluid is analyzed for percentage of fetal cells. One must remember that amniotic fluid contaminated by fetal blood will contain spuriously high levels of alpha-fetoprotein. Rarely do fetal cells comprise more than 5% of the total cells counted. However, we know from experience with placental aspiration that it is possible to obtain a significant percentage of fetal cells from a specimen of amniotic fluid without fetal jeopardy. It is theoretically possible, nonetheless, for a rent to be produced in a fetal vessel with a 20-gauge needle through which a significant percentage of fetal blood volume can be extruded. For this reason, it is probably safer to perform a genetic tap at about 16 weeks when 1 cc. of fetal blood would represent no more than a 6% blood volume depletion. The same 1 cc. blood loss would represent a 15% volume deficit to a 14-week fetus.

The morbidity in second trimester amniocenteses, reported in a recent collaborative study, is similar statistically to the expected incidence of second trimester abortion in the general population. Nonetheless, many investigators have noted morbidity to be temporally related to amniocentesis, and the above study should not lead the physician to perform amniocentesis with a cavalier attitude. The largest contributor to morbidity within a few days of the tap is labor leading to abortion. There is some suspicion that this may be a result of placental separation. Rupture of the membranes with ultimate abortion has also been described. In about 5% of cases, however, there is leakage of amniotic fluid per vagina, which ceases immediately or within a few days of the tap. We feel this does not represent frank rupture of the membranes but an extramembranous accumulation of fluid, which is expelled by the uterus. This is not an ominous sign, and the patient is not at greater risk of intrauterine infection because the membranes adjacent to the cervix are intact. Fetal death has been reported after amniocentesis and may be associated with a fetal bleed. It is frequently difficult to implicate the procedure when fetal death occurs many days after an amniocentesis, since the patients being tapped are often at risk for fetal problems.

Ideally, those requiring genetic diagnoses should be referred to a unit where the procedure is routinely carried out by a team skilled in the techniques of amniocentesis and performed in the ultrasound laboratory.

Third trimester amniocentesis

It seems that each month another report emerges about a new test performed on amniotic fluid which provides new information about the condition or maturity of the fetus. Rarely is mention made of better techniques to obtain this valuable fluid.

When ultrasound was not available, physicians would pick one of three general areas to tap:

1 over the fetal small parts
2 in the nuchal area
3 just above the symphysis

Since there is generally between 800 and 1200 cc. of amniotic fluid in late pregnancy, fluid can usually be found with "blind" insertion of a needle into one of the above areas. However, with such a technique there is no logical way to avoid the placenta, the umbilical cord, or certain fetal vital structures. For instance, although there is generally fluid to be found in the vicinity of the fetal limbs, one encounters the thickest portion of the placenta here, if it is anteriorly implanted. Also, if the nuchal area is chosen and the umbilical cord is around the neck of the fetus, it is immobile and cannot be pushed away from the needle as when it is freely floating.

It is for these reasons and others that morbidity can be lowered appreciably when ultrasound is utilized adjunctively in third trimester amniocentesis, since the operator is allowed the luxury of knowing the exact position of all the intrauterine contents.

The technique is similar to that described in the second trimester amniocentesis, in that a pocket of fluid away from the placenta is selected (Figure 4). If placental penetration is unavoidable, then it should not be penetrated in the area of the cord insertion.

Because of the relative immobility of the fetus in late gestation, it is extremely difficult, with the exception of a suprapubic amniocentesis, to create pockets of fluid by manipulating the fetus. One simply must search for the fluid. In oligohydramnios, we often have been successful in finding a small pocket of fluid just lateral to and below the fetal chin. This area, however, should never be used without ultrasonic localization, because of its proximity to the fetal face and neck. If no suitable accumulation of fluid can be demonstrated by ultrasound and a suprapubic tap is

Figure 4

Third trimester amniocentesis.
Amniocentesis needle pathway represented by graticule.

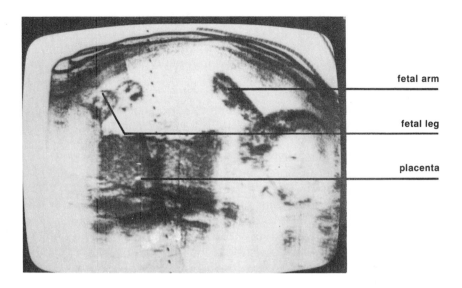

fetal arm

fetal leg

placenta

impossible, then the risks and benefits of the procedure must be reassessed. With experience, one learns not only where and when to tap but when *not* to tap.

The technique of needle insertion and fluid withdrawal is identical to that described above for the second trimester tap. If one wishes to tap laterally, it is often preferable to insert the needle medial to the fluid pocket and then direct the needle laterally once inside the amniotic cavity. With this method, the uterine vessels can be avoided. It must be remembered that because most uteri are dextrorotated, the vessels on the left are generally closer to the midline than those on the right. It must also be kept in mind that omentum or loops of bowel may be interposed between the top of the uterine fundus and the anterior abdominal wall; therefore, in the fundal tap the needle should be inserted into an area where the uterine fundus is in close approximation to the abdominal peritoneum.

If bloody fluid is obtained on insertion of the needle, the multiple syringe method can be utilized, and generally the fluid will clear. Once obtained, the fluid should be centrifuged and either analyzed immediately or frozen, with the exception of that obtained for spectrophotometric analysis. This fluid should be protected from light, maintained at a constant pH, and analyzed within a few hours.

Complications

The morbidity associated with third trimester amniocentesis is real, and with its expanded use emerge more reports of fetal pneumothorax, pneumomediastinum, umbilical cord hematoma, and fetal exsanguination. If bloody fluid is obtained and especially if the blood does not clear in the third syringe, the fetal heart rate should be monitored externally by Doppler or phonocardiogram. As in the second trimester tap, the fluid should be analyzed for percentage of fetal cells. This analysis may take 45 min., and the patient should not be discharged until the results are obtained. If more than 5% fetal cells are seen, the fetal heart rate should be monitored for at least 2 hr. If the fetal blood volume is depleted significantly by the procedure, the baseline fetal heart rate will gradually rise. If sensitive phonocardiographic or abdominal EKG equipment is available, then the beat-to-beat difference can be appreciated. A volume-depleted baby should exhibit a smooth heart rate. Rarely, if the cord has been manipulated or if a hematoma is developing in the cord or in its placental insertion, a precipitous drop in fetal heart rate will be noted. This is an ominous sign if it continues; and if the patient is at a stage in gestation where there is reasonable chance of extrauterine survival, an immediate cesarean section should be performed. Fortunately, these complications are rare, and the reader should be reassured by the fact that in the past 4 yr. of experience with this technique at Yale only one cesarean section has been performed for an amniocentesis-related complication.

Needle aspiration transducers

A- and B-mode amniocentesis transducers have been designed to aid the operator in directing a needle to a desired location in the intrauterine cavity. When passed through the central hole of the transducer, the tip of the needle emits an echo which is separate from echoes produced by other intrauterine structures. This phenomenon permits the physician to know where the needle tip is in relation to these structures.

We have found these transducers to be invaluable in special procedures such as fetoscopy and intrauterine transfusion. Its usefulness, however, in amniocentesis is somewhat limited because with needles of small gauge it is difficult to obtain a discernible echo using transducers that are currently on the market. This problem can be alleviated by diminishing the hole diameter and increasing transducer frequency. Some manufacturers are now working on this, and real-time B-mode aspiration transducers may also be available in the near future.

Indices of fetal condition

Amniotic fluid bilirubin (ΔOD) With the advent of antiimmune globulin, Rh disease is largely preventable. However, many patients were sensitized before this therapeutic modality became available, and reports are increasing of Rh sensitization because of insufficient dosage of anti-D globulin in patients with large fetomaternal transfusions at the time of delivery. Consequently, there are still patients with this dwindling disease to manage. Since maternal anti-D antibody crosses the placenta and reacts with the red cells of the fetus, which are then removed from the effective fetal circulation, the fetus becomes progressively anemic. It was noticed years ago that a portion of the bilirubin liberated from the breakdown of these cells appears as unconjugated bilirubin in the amniotic fluid. Relative amounts of the chloroform-soluble bilirubin can be appreciated in amniotic fluid because it has a characteristic spectral absorption at 450 mμ. The difference between the expected spectrophotometric curve of amniotic fluid at 450 mμ and that found in an Rh-affected patient (Figure 5), the ΔOD, is then plotted on a chart devised by Liley (Figure 6). The severity of the disease generally correlates with magnitude of the optical density difference.

With this information, it has been possible to decrease significantly mortality rates in Rh disease. It is a far more accurate way of following the fetal status than with serum anti-D titers alone, but it still is at best an indirect method. A variety of other factors may affect the amniotic fluid bilirubin level. Phenothiazines may increase the ΔOD, and phenobarbital may decrease it. A rise in maternal bilirubin will be reflected in the amniotic fluid level. Other pigments (oxyhemoglobin, meconium, conjugated bilirubin, etc.) sometimes interfere with the spectrophotometric interpretation; and light changes, temperature, and pH may also affect the ΔOD.

Figure 5

ΔOD: difference between optical density at 450 mμ in normal and Rh-affected amniotic fluid.

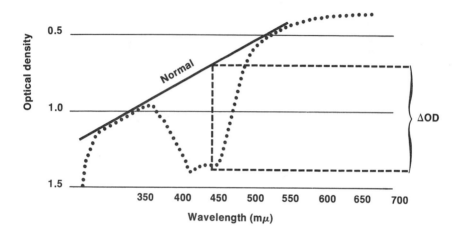

Figure 6

Logarithmic curve of OD throughout pregnancy indicating prognostic zones (Liley).

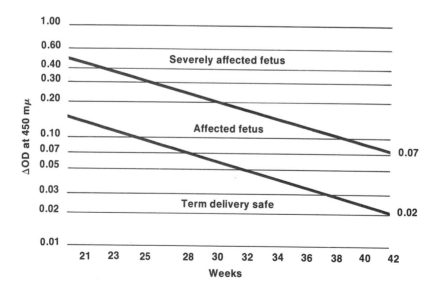

As indicated in another chapter, work is in progress to obtain safely fetal blood from a placental vessel in utero; and if and when this technique is perfected, it will be possible to follow the severity of fetal anemia by direct measurement of the fetal hematocrit.

Meconium For many years it has been known that meconium-stained amniotic fluid was often a sign of intrauterine jeopardy. There is no doubt that about 50% of distressed fetuses will pass meconium; but what are the chances of fetal distress if one unexpectedly finds meconium at amniocentesis or at rupture of membranes before labor? The question may be partially answered by reviewing the literature on amnioscopy. One investigator has noted a five-fold increase in perinatal mortality when meconium was found by amnioscopy prior to labor. It seems, however, that labor and delivery are the primary threat to the potentially compromised fetus residing in meconium-stained amniotic fluid. For instance, 1.7% of fetuses with this finding were acidotic preceding labor, while 31% of babies who had meconium staining prior to labor were acidotic at delivery, as determined by umbilical artery pH analysis. Since it is thought that meconium is passed as a result of anoxic insult and that labor statistically and logically is a stress to the fetus in jeopardy, it is not surprising that these babies often demonstrate fetal heart rate patterns of uteroplacental insufficiency when monitored in labor and are acidotic at birth. Although many papers have been written about meconium in amniotic fluid, it is very difficult to extract enough objective data to answer the questions that arise when one encounters this phenomenon.

Why does the fetus pass meconium? It has been supposed that either there is relaxation of the anal sphincter or increased peristalsis in the compromised fetus. This has been noted when the oxygen saturation drops below 30%. We have seen babies, however, that have very recently died in utero, and the amniotic fluid is clear, so this is not an all-or-none phenomenon. In some cases, meconium staining may simply be a chance finding that occurs throughout gestation as a result of an innocuous temporary impingement of the umbilical cord. Apparently, normal fetuses can pass meconium as early as the second trimester of pregnancy.

It seems that there is one obstetrical dilemma in which meconium-stained amniotic fluid is an excellent predictor of the fetal condition, and this is in the 3.5% of patients whose gestation has progressed beyond the 42nd week. About one out of 10 of these post-date patients will deliver babies with post-mature syndrome, and these babies are subject to significantly higher rates of mortality and morbidity. Since it is rare for the fetus with post-maturity syndrome not to have meconium staining, a finding of meconium-tinged fluid by amniocentesis in prolonged gestation is a definite sign of danger.

We feel that if meconium is found after rupture of membranes before or during labor, fetal heart rate monitoring is essential. If a patient whose pregnancy has progressed past the 42nd week has meconium-stained fluid at the time of an amniocentesis, labor should be induced immediately.

Although the appearance of meconium in a tap performed to ascertain maturity in the third trimester may just be a chance finding of innocuous consequences, there is still sufficient reason to perform an oxytocin challenge test to identify possible fetal compromise.

Indices of maturity

L/S ratio This test has been of tremendous value in the management of high risk pregnancies, elective inductions, and repeat cesarean sections. Recently, it has been found through the diligent work of many investigators that premature babies who are born without an ability to produce a surface-active phospholipid, dipalmitoyl lecithin, will develop the classic hyaline membrane disease (or the more appropriate term, respiratory distress syndrome, RDS). This phospholipid lines the alveoli and by lowering surface tension keeps the alveoli from collapsing after each expired breath. The resulting 40% residual air mass is essential in maintaining oxygen transfer in the neonate.

Since the fetal tracheal-bronchial tree contributes in part to the contents of the amniotic fluid, Gluck set about to prove that pulmonic maturity could be predicted in utero by analyzing amniotic fluid for the presence or absence of this material. In 1971, he first published a technique to measure relative amounts of lecithin and another phospholipid, sphingomyelin, in amniotic fluid by thin-layer chromatography. With this L/S ratio, he noted (Figure 7) that the lecithin is found in smaller amounts in early gestation than

Figure 7

Concentration of lecithin and sphingomyelin throughout gestation.

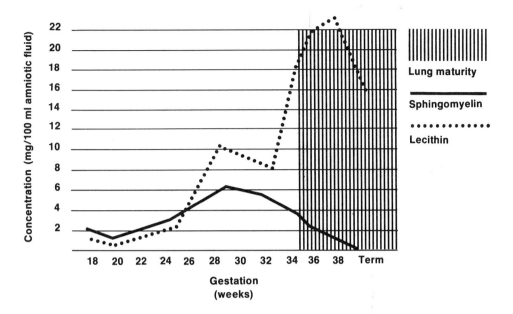

sphingomyelin; but that a ratio of 1:1 was attained at 32 weeks, and a ratio of 2:1 was generally noted after the 35th week of gestation. Babies born after a ratio of 2:1 did not develop RDS, while babies born after an intermediate tap (1:5 to 2:0) could develop RDS. Ratios of less than 1:5 were often associated with severe RDS and neonatal death.

The literature is now replete with reports of experience with this diagnostic test of pulmonic maturity. Many investigators, however, elected to modify the original technique; and it is now difficult to interpret the diverse results reported when a common technique is not utilized. However, we will try to summarize our experience and that of other investigators using the same L/S ratio technique.

A ratio of greater than 2 in over 95% of cases is associated with a baby that does not develop RDS. Most of the false positive L/S ratios reported have been in infants of diabetic mothers. In our experience of over 3 yr., we have had only three babies that developed mild to moderate RDS after a mature L/S ratio. They were all infants of diabetic mothers, and they all were asphyxic at the time of birth with low 5-min. Apgar scores.

In general, if an L/S ratio is less than 2, the infant has a 25% chance of developing RDS; but the lower the ratio by densitometric quantitation, the greater the chance of RDS.

Maternal blood contains lecithin; consequently, the L/S ratio may be affected by blood in the amniotic fluid. The lecithin concentration remains constant in maternal blood throughout gestation, and it has been demonstrated that only the intermediate ratio (1.5:2.0) is suspect after bloody taps because maternal blood will slightly diminish a ratio above 2 and will tend to minimally raise a ratio below 1.5. Therefore, ratios above 2 and below 1.5 should be valid even in traumatically obtained samples. The L/S ratio is not affected when the hematocrit of the fluid obtained is less than 1%. Meconium apparently binds lecithin, and this may also affect the L/S ratio.

A "bedside" test for pulmonic maturity, known by most as a "foam test," qualitatively predicts the presence or absence of surface-active phospholipids. Although disarmingly simple, it is not a bedside test and must be precisely performed. Reports have been somewhat conflicting concerning the correlation of this test with the L/S ratio and with the clinical condition of the neonate.

It should be mentioned that not all investigators are in accord that L/S ratio is specifically a measure of pulmonic maturity, and one author feels that the test correlates better with age and weight of the fetus than with the incidence of RDS.

Creatinine The fetal kidney begins functioning as early as 12 to 14 weeks gestation. At this time, excretion is exclusively by glomerular filtration. The fetal kidney develops tubular function at about the 24th week of gestation, and it is from this time on that the composition of amniotic fluid no longer resembles that of fetal serum. Glomerular filtration continues throughout gestation, and urine production increases as pregnancy progresses. Creatinine is filtered by the kidney, and its appearance in urine is a function of:

1 the amount of fetal body mass and
2 renal function.

There is no doubt that creatinine is excreted into the amniotic fluid, but the fetal kidney is not its exclusive source. There is a definite relationship between maternal serum creatinine levels and amniotic fluid concentrations of this breakdown product of muscle mass.

Creatinine levels rise as pregnancy progresses in a linear fashion until about the 34th week of gestation, when the concentration rises more acutely. In general, most studies indicate levels of about 2.0 mg. percent to be associated with mature fetuses in over 90% of cases. Levels below 1.5 mg. percent are generally noted when the fetus is premature. However, many variables can affect the creatinine concentration, producing false positive and negative results. Creatinine levels may be erroneously high in relative oligohydramnios or when maternal creatinine levels are high because of compromised maternal renal function. We have even noted false positive creatinine levels in patients in whom we could find no apparent reason for elevated values. Conditions such as intrauterine growth retardation, Rh disease, and diabetes can also be associated with falsely low creatinine levels. In general, fetuses compromised by the above diseases may have decreased renal plasma flow with a fall in glomerular filtration of creatinine. Recently, small-for-dates fetuses have been shown to produce less urine than normal fetuses for the same gestational age.

The benefit of amniotic fluid creatinine is best appreciated when it is used in conjunction with other tests of fetal maturity. If used alone, its usefulness diminishes.

Other indices of maturity

Orange cell count As the fetus matures, fat becomes incorporated into the cells of the skin. These cells are extruded into the amniotic fluid, and cells specifically sloughed from the adnexal glands will stain orange when amniotic fluid containing these cells is mixed with 0.1% Nile blue sulfate. These fat cells appear at about 32 to 34 weeks in the amniotic fluid, and at term approximately 50% of cells stained in this manner will contain fat. If the percentage of orange cells is less than 10, 85% of the babies will be premature. Initial reports indicated a very low percentage of premature babies to be associated with an orange cell count of over 20%, yet in a recent report 27% of babies with a mature orange cell count were, in fact, premature.

∆OD

It was noted in 1967 that about 75% of patients spontaneously began labor within 4 weeks of an amniotic fluid ∆OD of zero. Eighty-five percent of babies delivered after this reading weighed more than 6 lb. From these and other data, it was suggested that amniotic fluid bilirubin determinations would be good predictors of fetal maturity, because the absence of unconjugated bilirubin in amniotic fluid was probably a function of maturing fetal enzymatic activity. As pointed out, however, a variety of drugs can falsely elevate or lower the ∆OD, as will maternal changes in bilirubin. Even in the absence of these conditions, one author reports an incidence of false negativity of over 50% and false positivity of 10%.

Miscellaneous indices of fetal maturity

Other amniotic fluid parameters have been used to predict fetal age, such as osmolality, uric acid, urea, amylase. But either data are too scarce to make a judgment about their worth or, as in osmolality determinations, the scatter of points on a normal curve precludes precise interpretation.

Each of the above tests of maturity is telling us something different about the baby. Glucuronyl transferase activity may not coincide with maturation of the fetal kidney. Lung maturity may appear before 20% of extruded amniotic fluid cells contain fat. Consequently, a combination of the above tests will definitely correlate better with gestational age of the fetus than one analysis alone. It must be remembered, however, that the most common cause of death in the premature infant is RDS; and if it can be predicted in utero by an L/S ratio that a baby will not develop this disease, the importance of the other tests must be put in perspective.

Amniocentesis and the future

As techniques and analyses develop, amniotic fluid may provide even more information about the fetus and its intrauterine environment. There may be certain clues in amniotic fluid, such as levels of hydroxyproline, which may assist in identifying the fetus that is undergoing intrauterine malnutrition. Aspiration of the fluid is already helpful in diagnosing early amnionitis when bacteria are found in the specimen.

Amniotic fluid may also become an invaluable vehicle to deliver nutrients and medications in situations where it is necessary to circumvent the placenta. We know that the fetus will normally swallow as much as 1 gram of protein per day, and it has the enzymatic capability to digest certain proteins and amino acids. In cases where placental transfer of nutrients is impaired, as in toxemia or chronic hypertension, alimentation could be accomplished by the deposition of nutrients into the amniotic cavity. Some substances, such as tri-iodothyronine (T_3) and thyroxin (T_4), normally traverse the placenta in negligible amounts. In cases where there is the possibility of cretinism, thyroid hormone could be delivered to the fetus through the amniotic fluid to insure normal mental development. Obviously, careful investigative studies must be initiated before this can be used clinically.

Fetoscopy and fetal blood sampling

Although the availability of amniotic fluid has been responsible for recent progress in prenatal genetic diagnosis, there are limitations to what information this fluid can provide. Of the cells extruded into amniotic fluid, 90% are dead or dying, and the fluid itself does not express all the metabolic functions of the fetus. Therefore, some investigators have recently attempted to view the fetus, obtain fetal skin biopsies, and sample its blood. All these procedures are accomplished through a small endoscope and specially designed cannula for fetal blood drawing.

As in amniocentesis, the technique requires ultrasound. Perhaps the most important step in the fetoscopic method is the selection of the abdominal insertion site. The exact position of the fetus is delineated with ultrasound. If the operator wishes to sample blood from a posterior placenta, then the endoscope is inserted over the area of the fetal limbs so there will be unobstructed access to the placenta (see Figure 3). If the fetal back is to be examined, an insertion site is chosen over the fetal spine. We have found the needle aspiration transducer to be extremely useful in the technique. The tip of the cannula housing the endoscope emits an echo on the oscilloscope, which is separate from other intra-abdominal echoes (Figure 8), as the cannula is passed through the central hole of the transducer, which lies on the patient's abdomen. This allows the operator to know exactly where the endoscope is within the uterine cavity. The endoscopes being used

Figure 8a

Actual A-mode ultrasonograph.

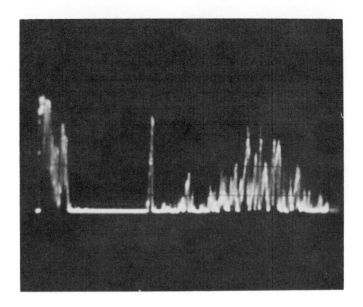

are extremely small, and the visual field is narrowed appreciably by the magnification imposed by the small diameter of the endoscope (about the size of a 16-gauge needle).

If a skin biopsy is to be obtained from the fetal scalp, the needle aspiration transducer becomes even more important. The technique we use requires that the endoscope be removed from the cannula after a biopsy site on the fetal scalp is selected visually. Since at our best optic distance the endoscope is only a few millimeters away from the object viewed, it is easy to maneuver the cannula and biopsy forceps within the cannula the remaining distance to the scalp. Resistance is encountered when the cannula echo and the scalp echo merge on the A-mode oscilloscope. Fetal movement during the "blind period" can be appreciated ultrasonically, and the procedure is started again.

Since fetal blood provides specific information about genetically transmitted diseases, especially hemoglobinopathies such as sickle cell anemia and thalassemia, two techniques have been developed to obtain this blood. Ultrasound plays an integral part in both methods.

Figure 8b
Aminocentesis technique.

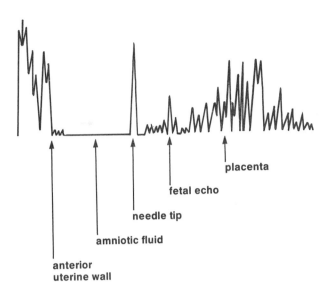

Figure 8c
Schematic representation of sagittal section through the uterus.
Technique of fetoscopy using needle aspiration
transducer.

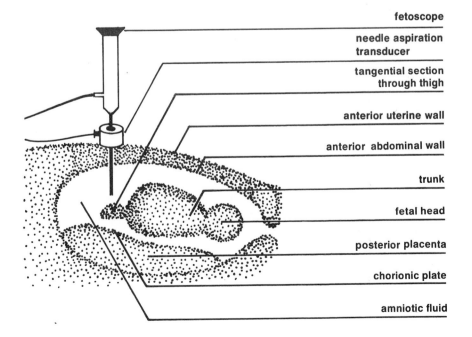

Figure 9

Schematic representation of fetal blood drawing.

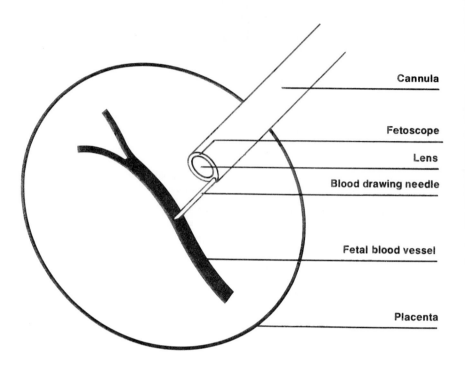

Cannula

Fetoscope

Lens

Blood drawing needle

Fetal blood vessel

Placenta

Using fetoscopy, it is possible to visualize blood vessels on the placental surface which contain fetal blood. A cannula has been designed with a Y side arm. When an endoscope is inserted into the cannula, a channel is created alongside the endoscope allowing passage of a 27-gauge needle. After a suitable placental vessel is selected visually, the 27-gauge needle is inserted into the Y side arm, advanced through the channel next to the endoscope, and directed into the placental vessel (Figure 9). Blood is drawn up into a syringe attached to the hub of the 27-gauge needle. With this method, it has been possible to obtain a suitable sample of blood for hemoglobin analysis in 96% of second trimester patients with posterior placentas. In some patients with anterior placentas, it has been possible with ultrasound to direct the endoscope through the placenta to sample blood from a low-lying lateral or fundal extension of the placenta.

Since no short-term ill-effects were noted in mother or fetus after fetoscopy and fetal blood sampling in patients about to undergo elective abortion, and since it has been possible to study globin chain synthesis in this blood, the procedure is now being offered to patients at risk for delivering babies with sickle cell disease or beta-thalassemia. To date, 17 patients have been studied. Ten have delivered without event, five elected to abort when studies indicated the fetus had beta-thalassemia, and the remaining pregnancies are progressing normally.

Placental aspiration

Fetal blood can also be obtained by placental aspiration. To our knowledge, Frederick Frigoletto was the first to attempt to obtain fetal blood by directing a needle into the placental substance. Kan and Valenti first reported their ability to obtain fetal blood with this technique. They were able to obtain enough fetal blood for hemoglobin analysis in 11 of 19 patients who were to have therapeutic abortions. Although some 12 continuing pregnancies have been studied by placental aspiration by Golbus and Kan, many more procedures will have been performed by the time this text is published.

The technique is relatively simple. The placenta is localized and the margins clearly delineated with gray scale. We have found higher frequency transducers (3.5, 5 MHz) to be invaluable in displaying placental architecture, especially in anterior placentas. Then, either using a high frequency needle aspiration transducer with a small hole or by reference to the displayed video picture, a 20-gauge spinal needle is directed to a location where the tip is just inside the chorionic plate, where 0.1 to 0.3 ml. of blood is aspirated into a heparinized syringe. Many small samples are then obtained at different levels within the placenta, and a sample is also obtained from amniotic fluid adjacent to the punctured placenta. These samples will contain between 0% and 80% fetal blood. One must obtain at *least* 5% fetal cells for hemoglobin studies. The maternal blood obtained is undoubtedly from the intravillous space, and the fetal blood must be coming from traumatized fetal cotyledons.

The comparative efficiency of obtaining fetal blood and the relative risks to the fetus and pregnancy of endoscopic sampling versus placental aspiration should become known in the future. At this point, however, it should be mentioned that because of the progress in ultrasonic imagery, coupled with the limitations of endoscopic visualization, ultrasound should eclipse the use of fetoscopy in the prediction of congenital anomalies such as limb, cranial, and spine defects.

Abortion

It is not within the design of this text to deal with the ethics of abortion. It would suffice to say that patients in many countries can now legally seek to have their pregnancies terminated, and it is the responsibility of doctors asked to perform these abortions to use the best techniques that will insure the safety of these patients.

Abortions are performed until fetal viability is attained. Viability means an ability of a fetus to sustain extrauterine life, but there seems to be no common definition of when that occurs. To some, this extrauterine life starts at 24 weeks or 500 grams; to others, 20 weeks. Therefore, the point in gestation beyond which abortion cannot be performed varies between hospitals. The easiest time to interrupt a pregnancy is in the first trimester. This is basically accomplished by dilating the cervix to accommodate cannulas of varying thicknesses, and the products of conception are removed by suction curettage.

Suction curettage may be performed safely until the 12th week of gestation, after which there is an increased incidence of hemorrhage, retained products of conception with resulting infection, and perforation. Although most physicians are unwilling to perform suction curettage after the 12th week of gestation, in about 5% of cases the patient's dates are inaccurate and/or the examiner fails to appreciate the size of the uterus on pelvic exam. In these cases, the physician is confronted with the dangerous task of emptying a uterus which is more than 12 weeks' size by suction curettage.

This pitfall can be overcome with the judicious use of ultrasound. For instance, if a patient is difficult to examine because of obesity, uterine retroversion, or because she is unable to relax during the examination, then the pregnancy can be dated with one scan. If the patient's dates indicate her pregnancy to be more than 12 weeks and the pelvic exam suggests an 11- or 12-week gestation, a scan would clear up the discrepancy between dates and the sometimes fallible pelvic exam.

In the second trimester abortion where the uterine fundus is at or above the umbilicus, a scan is helpful in distinguishing the viable from the non-viable pregnancy. Many institutions will permit abortion only when the BPD is below a predetermined figure.

On occasion, we have localized retained products of conception with ultrasound in patients with post-abortion bleeding. If small amounts of tissue are present, however, it is difficult to distinguish this from decidua. In the second trimester abortion, it is often necessary to direct the needle into the amniotic cavity with ultrasound when physicians have been unable to inject prostaglandin or saline. The technique is identical to that described in the chapter on amniocentesis, and with it we have never failed to enter the cavity. Two patients in whom it was impossible to obtain amniotic fluid at the time of abortion were subsequently found to have hydatidiform moles by ultrasound.

Ideally, all second trimester abortion patients should have a scan and tap in the ultrasound lab, but this is impractical in a busy abortion service. If, however, a physician fails after one or two attempts to enter the cavity, there is sufficient reason to then employ ultrasound. Low cost portable real-time machines would be extremely useful because the scans and procedure could be carried out at the patient's bedside.

Intrauterine transfusion

Although the incidence of Rh-sensitized pregnancies is diminishing, some centers are still confronted with patients whose fetuses are affected with severe erythroblastosis fetalis. When amniotic fluid studies indicate that demise is imminent in a fetus too premature to be delivered, then an intrauterine transfusion has been utilized as a life-saving procedure. Since its inception, the technique of intrauterine transfusion required the use of x-ray to localize the fetal peritoneal cavity and image intensification for localization of the tip of the transfusing needle. Therefore, some fetuses have been exposed to large amounts of x-ray radiation, especially when repeated transfusions were required.

A new method utilizing ultrasound has been designed to minimize fetal radiation and to allow the physician more control in placing the needle in the peritoneal cavity of the fetus.

By scanning sagittally and transversely, one can choose a penetration site on the maternal abdomen that will allow direct access to an entry point in the fetal peritoneal cavity between the level of the bladder and the umbilicus (Figure 10). The distance between the maternal abdominal wall and the middle of the fetal cavity (which is designated by an electronic marker on the A-mode oscilloscope) is recorded (Figure 11). The transfusing needle is then inserted through the central hole of an A-mode needle aspiration transducer and advanced until the echo from the tip of the needle is over the electronic marker. One can determine that the needle tip is in proper position by injecting a water-soluble radiopaque medium through the needle. With a few seconds of image intensification, the injected solution can be seen to pass between loops of fetal bowel. The transfusion is accomplished by injecting packed red blood cells through the transfusing needle.

Provided with instantaneous ultrasonic information, one is more secure in knowing where the tip of the transfusing needle is in relation to certain fetal vital structures. One author (F.W.) has recently used real-time examination alone for intrauterine transfusion successfully in six cases. The needle could be observed to enter the fetal abdomen, and the entire injection was monitored with ultrasound. This was accomplished by placing the real-time transducer adjacent to the needle at an angle of about 30 degrees.

After completion of the interperitoneal transfusion, the fetal abdomen can be scanned to verify that the fluid has been introduced into the peritoneal cavity.

Figure 10a

Midline sagittal section illustrating position of transducer and needle in intrauterine transfusion.
Tip of needle is in the middle of the fetal abdominal cavity. *Dotted line* extending from needle tip indicates the scanning angle in transverse section in Figure 10*b*.

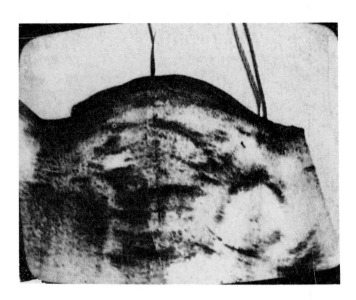

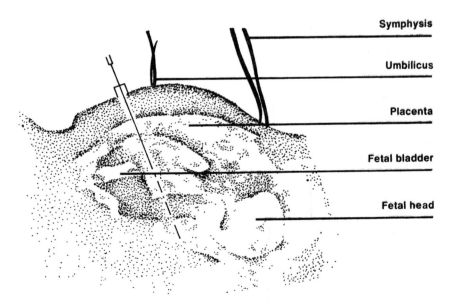

Symphysis

Umbilicus

Placenta

Fetal bladder

Fetal head

Figure 10b

Transverse section at level of needle insertion site.
Needle and transducer schematically represented.
Needle tip in peritoneal cavity.

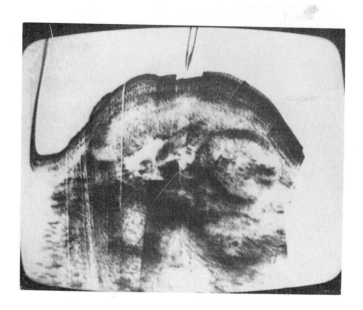

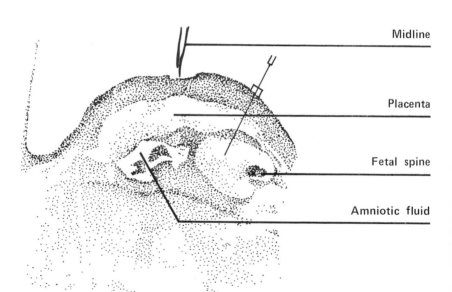

Midline

Placenta

Fetal spine

Amniotic fluid

Figure 11

A-mode representation of maternal and fetal echoes.

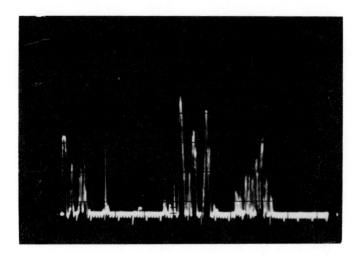

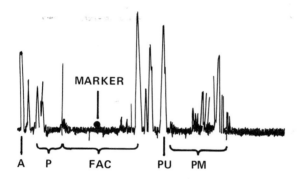

References

1 **Alter, B.P., Modell, C.B., Hobbins, J.C., et al.** Experience with antenatal detection of hemoglobinopathies. N. Engl. J. Med., 295:26, 1976.

2 **Bang, A.** A new ultrasonic method for transabdominal amniocentesis. Am. J. Obstet. Gynecol. 114:599, 1972.

3 **Bartsch, P.K., Lundberg, J., and Wahlstrom, J.** The technique, results and risks of amniocentesis for genetic reasons. J. Obstet. Gynaecol. Br. Commonw. 81:991, 1974.

4 **Brosens, I., and Gordon, H.** Estimation of maturity by cytological examination of liquor amnii. J. Obstet. Gynaecol. Br. Commonw. 73:118, 1966.

5 **Chang, H., Hobbins, J.C., Cividalli, G., Frigoletto, F.D., Mahoney, M.J., Kan, Y.W., and Nathan, D.G.** In utero diagnosis of hemoglobinopathies. Hemoglobin synthesis in fetal red cells. N. Engl. J. Med. 290:1067, 1974.

6 **Cooke, L.N., Shott, R.J., and Andrews, B.F.** Pediatrics 53:421, 1974.

7 **Curtis, J.D., Cohen, W.N., Richerson, H.B., and White, C.A.** The importance of placental localization preceding amniocentesis. Obstet. Gynecol. 40:194, 1972.

8 **Dallaire, L., Pinsky, L., Kinch, R.A., and Winsberg, F.** Prenatal diagnosis in medical genetics. Union Med. Can. 100:2213, 1971.

9 **Gluck, L., et al.** Diagnosis of respiratory distress syndrome (RDS) by amniocentesis. Am. J. Obstet. Gynecol. 109:440, 1971.

10 **Gluck, L., and Kulovich, M.V.** Lecithin/sphingomyelin ratios in amniotic fluid in normal and abnormal pregnancy. Am. J. Obstet. Gynecol. 115:539, 1973.

11 **Goldberg, B.B., and Pollack, A.M.** Ultrasonic aspiration-biopsy transducer. Radiology 108:667, 1973.

12 **Grove, C.S., Trombetta, G.C., and Amstey, M.S.** Fetal complications of amniocentesis. Am. J. Obstet. Gynecol. 115:1154, 1973.

13 **Hobbins, J.C.** Clinical experience with fetoscopy and fetal blood sampling. In *Intrauterine Fetal Visualization: A Multidisciplinary Approach,* edited by M. A. Kaback and C. Valenti. American Elsevier Publishing Co., Inc., New York, 1976.

14 **Hobbins, J.C., Davis, C.D., and Webster, J.** A new technique utilizing ultrasound to aid in intrauterine transfusion. J. Clin. Ultrasound 4:135, 1976.

15 **Hobbins, J.C., and Mahoney, M.J.** Experience with fetal blood drawing. Lancet 2:107, 1975.

16 **Hobbins, J.C., and Mahoney, M.J.** Experience with fetoscopy and fetal blood drawing. In *Endoscopy,* edited by G. Berci. Appleton-Century Crofts, New York, 1976.

17 **Hobbins, J.C., and Mahoney, M.J.** Fetoscopy and fetal blood sampling: the present state of the method. In *Clinical Obstetrics & Gynecology,* edited by H.J. Osofsky. Harper & Row, New York, 1975.

18 **Hobbins, J.C., and Mahoney, M.J.** In utero diagnosis of hemoglobinopathies. Technic for obtaining fetal blood. N. Engl. J. Med. 290:1065, 1974.

19 **Hobbins, J.C., Mahoney, M.J., and Goldstein, L.A.** New method of intrauterine evaluation by the combined use of fetoscopy and ultrasound. Am. J. Obstet. Gynecol. 118:1069, 1974.

20 **Hobel, C.J.** Intrapartum clinical assessment of fetal distress. Am. J. Obstet. Gynecol. 110:336, 1971.

21 **Jung, H., Kopecky, P., and Abramowski, P.** Ultrasonic observations after our special technique of intrauterine transfusion. Ann. Ostet. Ginecol. Med. Perinat. 92:570, 1971.

22 **Leake, R.D., Hobel, C.J., and Lachman, R.S.** Neonatal pneumothorax and subcutaneous emphysema secondary to diagnostic amniocentesis. Obstet. Gynecol. 43:884, 1974.

23 **Levi, S.** Diagnostic use of ultrasonics in abortion. A study of 250 patients. Int. J. Gynaecol. Obstet. 11:195, 1973.

24 **Mahoney, M.J., and Hobbins, J.C.** Ultrasound and growth of amniotic-fluid cells. Lancet 2:454, 1973.

25 **Mandelbaum, B., Lacroix, G.G., and Robinson, A.R.** Determination of fetal maturity by spectrophotometric analysis of amniotic fluid. Obstet. Gynecol. 29:471, 1967.

26 **Milunsky, A. (Editorial).** Risk of amniocentesis for prenatal diagnosis. N. Engl. J. Med. 932, 1975.

27 **Miskin, M., Doran, J.A., Rudd, N., Gardner, H.A., Liedgren, S., and Benzie, R.** Use of ultrasound for placental localization in genetic amniocentesis. Obstet. Gynecol. 43:872, 1974.

28 **O'Leary, J.A ., and Bezjian, A.A.** Amniotic fluid fetal maturity score. Obstet. Gynecol. 38:375, 1971.

29 **Pitkin, R.M., and Zwirch, S.J.** Amniotic fluid creatinine. Am. J. Obstet. Gynecol. 98:1135, 1967.

30 **Robinson, H.P.** Sonar in the management of abortion. J. Obstet. Gynaecol. Br. Commonw. 79:90, 1972.

31 **Roux, J.F., Nakamura, J., and Brown, E.G.** Further observations on the determination of gestational age by amniotic fluid analysis. Am. J. Obstet. Gynecol. 116:633, 1973.

Gynecology

8

In the section on the complications of early pregnancy, some conditions which may be confused with gynecological problems were discussed. These include ectopic gestation and tumors associated with early pregnancy. The diagnostic problems of pelvic inflammatory disease and pelvic abscess were also discussed.

One of the fundamental problems in assessing pelvic masses is the decision as to whether they are cystic or solid. This distinction should be made accurately; in addition, gray scale technique can provide more subtle information.

In order to understand the criteria for the differentiation of cystic and solid masses, one must go back to the physical principles of ultrasound. The attenuation of sound by water is negligible. Therefore, a beam of sound which traverses water regains its energy upon encountering the strong interface between the posterior limit of the fluid collection and the solid tissue behind it. The interface produces a very strong reflection, and the echo reverberates in the tissue behind the fluid or cystic mass, resulting in a tail of dense echoes (Figure 1). A second feature of the truly cystic mass is that it contains no internal acoustic interfaces, i.e., the acoustic impedance of all the material within the cyst is identical. No echoes are produced within this volume of homogeneous acoustic impedance, even if high amplification settings are used. A third feature, based on anatomical configuration, is that cyst walls are smooth and well defined. It is more difficult to assess the anterior wall because of reverberation between its interface and the tissue in front of it. This phenomenon tends to produce some apparent internal echoes in the cyst, as it does in any fluid-containing organ (such as the urinary bladder) or the uterus containing amniotic fluid. With experience, reverberating echoes can be recognized.

Figure 1a
Large ovarian cyst filling most of abdominal cavity (white on black).

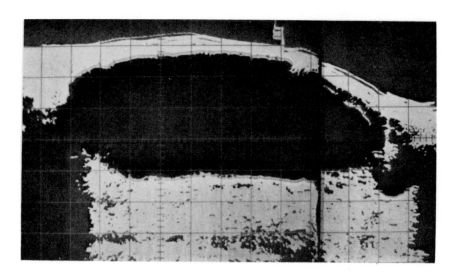

Figure 1b
A-mode representation of cyst.

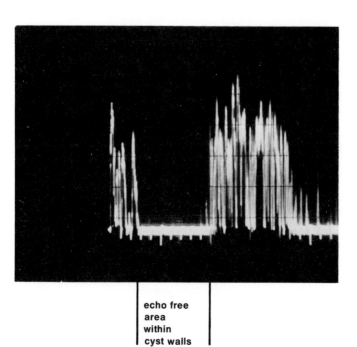

**echo free
area
within
cyst walls**

A fourth feature of the cyst, as distinguished from the solid tumor, is that if one changes to a higher frequency transducer, good penetration and demonstration of the posterior wall will be maintained. For this reason, it is useful to use 3.5 or 5 MHz transducers in the evaluation of pelvic masses. When scanning tumors of the thyroid and breast, we go as high as 10 MHz since they may be relatively small, and even when solid their attenuation at 2 MHz is minimal.

In the pelvis, the bladder is available as a standard of transonicity.

As one proceeds along the scale from cystic to solid, one encounters a group of conditions in which the acoustic attenuation is not as low as it is in the cyst but is not as high as it is in the solid tumor. These include hematomas, abscesses, and collections of blood such as one might encounter in an endometrioma (chocolate cyst). These masses may be distinguished from simple cysts by their relatively irregular wall outlines and the fact that they may contain some internal echoes produced by clotted blood, pus, or detritus (Figure 2). Further along this spectrum are the mixed cystic and solid masses. These include ovarian tumors which contain some solid elements such as pseudomucinous cystadenoma, pseudomucinous cystadenocarcinoma, and cystic teratomas containing solid elements such as hair and teeth. Cystic teratomas (dermoids) contain large quantities of fat (sebaceous material). X-ray studies of standing patients with dermoids have demonstrated the layering of this fat over cyst fluid, producing a sharp fat-fluid interface. This observation has also been made ultrasonically in patients with cystic teratomas of the ovary.

The next mass to be considered in this spectrum of relative densities is the leiomyoma of the uterus (Figure 3). Many fibroids are surprisingly transonic. As was mentioned in an earlier chapter, this is particularly true when they have undergone estrogenic stimulation and consequent edema or necrosis. Exogenous hormones can stimulate fibromyomas to undergo similar changes in the absence of pregnancy. We have observed huge transonic fibromyomas in young women taking oral contraceptive medication. Generally, fibroids are identified in relation to the adjacent uterus and are seen as bulges in its contour. Since they may contain calcium or other dense tissue, some of their tomographic slices will usually contain strong

Figure 2

Pelvic abscess.
Predominantly echo-free.
Note ragged border.

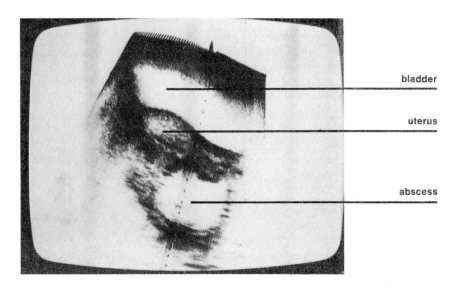

bladder

uterus

abscess

Figure 3

Leiomyoma of uterus.

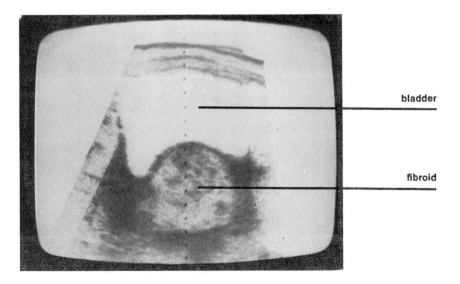

bladder

fibroid

echoes. Unlike cysts, the posterior borders of fibromyomas are rarely sharply delineated, and they do not show the tailing effect produced by the strong reverberation at the fluid-solid interface. If they are examined with higher frequency transducers, the posterior border will be only barely delineated.

Solid ovarian tumors must be differentiated from uterine leiomyomas. In general, it is useful to identify the uterus, and it may be possible to distinguish an extrauterine solid tumor from a fibroma if a clear outline of the displaced uterine cavity can be obtained. However, in the presence of large tumors, the uterus can be displaced so far away from its usual location that it may not be visible in the same scanning plane as the mass.

Pelvic inflammatory disease

Pelvic inflammatory disease is a common condition referred for ultrasonic examination. Pelvic abscesses are relatively easy to see. They displace the uterus and are usually closely adherent to the uterine wall. The uterus should be small, and at least one sagittal scan will show the small uterine cavity displaced by the relatively transonic but irregular mass. Another manifestation of pelvic inflammatory disease is the enlarged fallopian tube (hydrosalpinx). This is difficult to distinguish from a small ovarian cyst except that it tends to be elongated (Figure 4). In older patients, a pelvic abscess may be the result of diverticular disease, and its appearance is not distinguishable from a pelvic abscess due to primary pelvic inflammatory disease. Although some authors have reported increased echoes around the uterus resulting from adhesions, we do not believe that this is a reliable finding. Certainly, displacement of the uterus may accompany pelvic inflammatory disease without the demonstration of a mass, but even in a normal patient the uterus is frequently displaced to one side.

The ultrasonic examination will not demonstrate a mass in many patients who are clinically suspected of harboring one. The failure to demonstrate a mass is a significant negative finding in that it means that no cystic ovarian tumor, solid ovarian tumor, or abscess is present. In these patients, the palpable finding may be due to adhesions either resulting from inflammatory or bowel disease, or may be due to infiltrating metastatic tumor.

Figure 4
Hydrosalpinx.
Transverse scan.

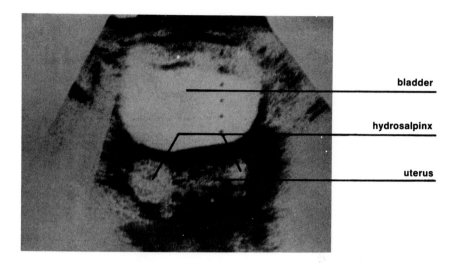

bladder

hydrosalpinx

uterus

The problem of ectopic pregnancy has already been discussed in an earlier chapter. This is a relatively common complication of pelvic inflammatory disease and is considered in the differential diagnosis of pelvic abscess.

Ovarian cysts

With ultrasonic equipment, which has high resolution and dynamic range, small cysts can be identified.

The cystic follicle, which is under 2 cm. in size, is sometimes seen. These thin walled structures contain clear serous fluid; they, therefore, have a markedly sonotranslucent appearance with very well defined walls. Ultrasound has proved helpful for the clinician in following the progression and retrogression of physiological cystic follicles.

Corpus luteum cysts are thicker walled and tend to be larger than follicle cysts but do not differ in appearance ultrasonically from follicle cysts. They are commonly seen with pregnancy and can be present in either ectopic or intrauterine gestations. A ruptured corpus luteum cyst simulates a ruptured ectopic pregnancy clinically and ultrasonically.

Figure 5

Multiloculated dermoid cyst.
Calcification is seen to produce acoustic shadow through cyst.

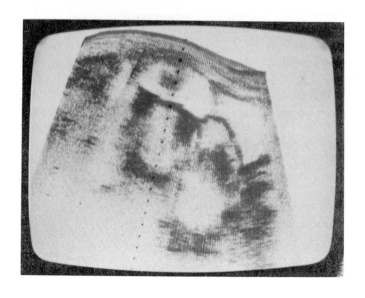

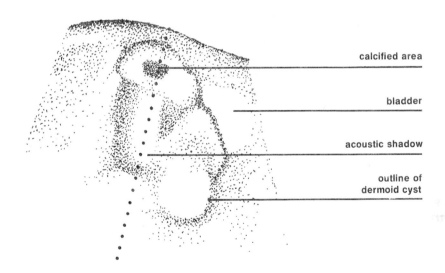

calcified area

bladder

acoustic shadow

outline of
dermoid cyst

Figure 6
Large dermoid cyst filling abdomen.

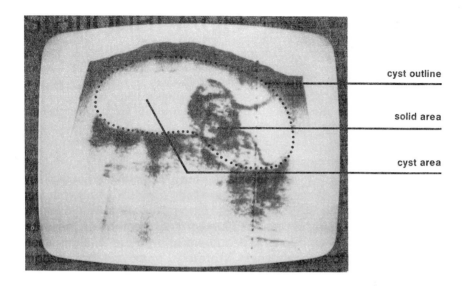

cyst outline

solid area

cyst area

The theca lutein cysts are the least common of the physiological cysts and are usually associated with trophoblastic tumors.

Paraovarian cysts are not distinguishable from ovarian cysts, and they may attain very large dimensions.

As was mentioned earlier, the dermoid cyst falls into the group of mixed cystic and solid lesions. Their ultrasonic appearance is extremely variable depending upon the gross pathological constituents. When they contain calcified material or hair, there may be acoustic shadowing within the tumor; and, in some cuts, the posterior wall of the cyst is eclipsed. When the diagnosis of the dermoid cyst is suspected, it is wise in the non-pregnant patient to obtain a radiograph of the abdomen for confirmation (Figures 5 and 6).

Solid teratomas of the ovary have no specific ultrasonic appearance.

Figure 7
Papillary cystadenocarcinoma.

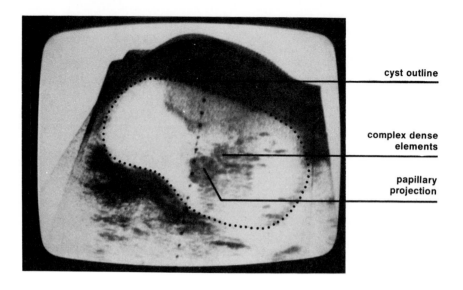

cyst outline

complex dense
elements

papillary
projection

Figure 8
Large pseudomucinous cystadenocarcinoma.
Complex echo pattern produced by loculation and mucinous
contour of cyst.

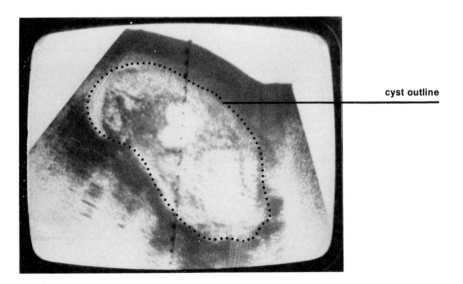

cyst outline

Serous cystomas of the ovary are non-specific in their appearance, resembling large physiological cysts or paraovarian cysts. Although they are commonly bilateral, the overlap of the two sides is such that the bilaterality is difficult to appreciate with ultrasound.

Cystadenomas may contain fibrous and adenomatous elements by gross pathological examination; therefore, it is not surprising that difficulty is encountered in ultrasonically distinguishing them from cystadenocarcinomas. The more irregular the wall of a cyst and complex the internal echo pattern, the more likely one is dealing with a malignant tumor (Figure 7).

Pseudomucinous cystadenomas are less common than serous cystadenomas. They tend to be multiloculated, and the mucinous content of some of the cysts increases the complexity of the echo pattern (Figure 8). They also may attain very large size and fill the entire abdominal cavity.

Ovarian malignancies may produce ascites, and this intraperitoneal fluid can be demonstrated in the pelvic flanks. When it is extensive, it can also be demonstrated lateral, inferior, and superior to the liver. In the presence of massive ascites, there are loops of bowel floating around in the pelvis, and these should not be mistaken for tumor masses. With real-time equipment their characteristic motion and gas transmission can be observed. Although some authors have described the differences between benign and malignant ascites, we do not believe that that differentiation is reliable.

As was stressed in the beginning of this book, the visualization of the pelvic organs requires a full bladder. It is futile to examine a patient with an empty bladder. However, occasionally, a large cystic mass cannot be definitely distinguished from the bladder. In that instance, the patient can be asked to void after the initial examination, and the cystic mass can then be differentiated from it.

Ultrasound appearance
of pelvic masses

Category According to Basic Ultrasound Appearance	Neoplastic	Diagnosis	Malignant	Specific Ultrasonic Qualites
1. Completely cystic	Rare	From follicle		
		Follicle cyst	No	
		Corpus luteum cyst		Completely cystic with smooth walls
		Corpus albicans cyst		
		From hilar remnants		
		Rete ovarii		
		Paratubal cyst		
		From surface epithelium		
		Single or multiple inclusion cyst		
		Neoplastic		
		Serous cystadenoma		
		Mucinous cystadenoma		Sometimes more solid components are noted
2. Cystic with solid pole possible	Possible	Cystic teratoma (dermoid)	Rare	Calcifications presenting as irregular densities within cyst; outline generally well defined but sometimes thick
		Endometriosis	No	Irregularly enlarged ovaries; fibrosis responsible for heterogeneous appearance; endometrioma sometimes appears as a mostly cystic adnexal mass
		Benign epithelial lesion (serous papillary cystoma) rare	No	Mostly cystic mass with intracystic solid areas

**Ultrasound appearance
of pelvic masses —**
continued

Category According to Basic Ultrasound Appearance	Neoplastic	Diagnosis	Malignant	Specific Ultrasonic Qualities
3. Cystic lesions with intrauterine papillary projections	Yes	Serous papillary cystoma	No	Broad based stromal polyps projecting into cyst; rather smooth walls
		Papillary serous cystadenocarcinoma	Yes	
		Endometrioid carcinoma	Yes	Irregular outline; intracystic projections
		Clear-cell carcinoma	Yes	
		Mucinous cystadenocarcinoma	Yes	
4. Solid lesions with cystic areas	Yes	Adenofibromas (mucinous cystadenoma) (Brenner tumor with mucinous component)	No	Cystic spaces within mostly solid, smooth walled tumor
	Yes	Necrosis and hemorrhage in any mostly solid malignant tumor where torsion occurs or blood supply outgrown	Yes	Irregular heterogeneous mass with cystic areas within; clot sometimes can be identified with gray scale
5. Solid lesions	Yes	Carcinoma (serous) — epithelial origin	Yes	Thick wall; irregular outline
		Fibroma — stromal origin	No	
	Yes	Leiomyoma	No	Solid homogeneous appearance
		Granulosa-cell tumor	Possible	
		Thecoma	No	
		Brenner	Rare	

References

1 **Buttery, B.W.** Ultrasonic hysterography. A new technique. Lancet 2:652, 1974.

2 **Kobayashi, M., Hellman, L.M., and Cromb, E.** *Atlas of Ultrasonography in Obstetrics and Gynecology,* Ed. 7, Appleton-Century-Crofts, New York, 1972.

3 **Morley, P., and Barnett, E.** The use of ultrasound in the diagnosis of pelvic masses. Br. J. Radiol. 43:602, 1970.

4 **Scheer, K., and Goldstein, D.P.** Use of ultrasonography to follow regression of theca lutein cysts. Radiology 108:673, 1973.

5 **von Micsky, L.I.** Gynecologic ultrasonography. *Diagnostic Ultrasound,* edited by D.L. King, pp. 207–241. C.V. Mosby Co., St. Louis, 1974.

Appendix

This appendix has been included to assist the reader in rapidly determining fetal age and weight and placental size from a variety of published formulas. We have also included a formula for fetal urine production.

Figure 1

Uterine volume: formula = length × width × thickness × 0.5233
(see Chapter 6).

From Gohari, P., Berkowitz, R.L., and Hobbins, J. C.: Prediction
of intrauterine growth retardation by determination of total intrauterine volume. Am. J. Obstet. Gynecol. 127:255, 1977.

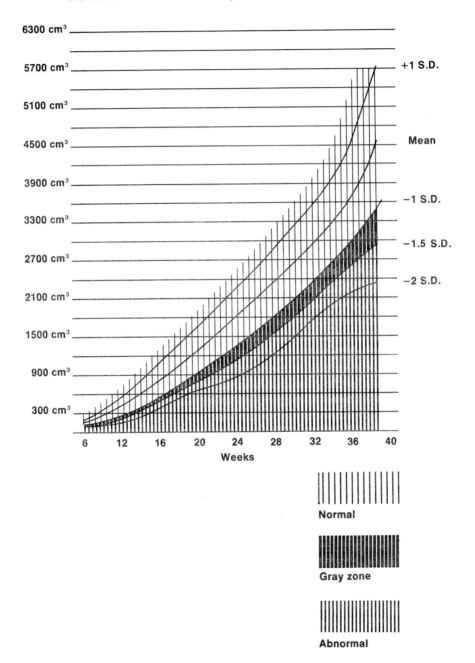

Figure 2

Placental growth curve. Volume determined by formula for planoconvex volume.

$$V = \frac{\pi}{6} \times h \left(\tfrac{3}{4} D_L D_T + h^2 \right)$$

From Hellman, L.M., Kobayashi, M., Tolles, W.E., and Cromb, E.: Ultrasonic studies on the volumetric growth of the human placenta. Am. J. Obstet. Gynec. 108:740–750, 1970.

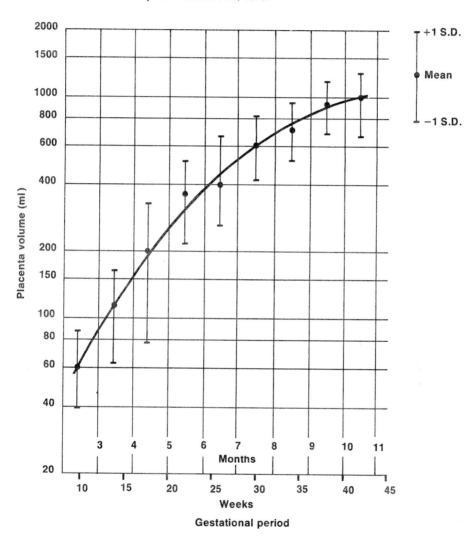

Gestational period

Figure 3

Mean values and scatter of results of 214 measurements of fetal crown-rump lengths from 6 to 14 weeks of menstrual age.

From Robinson, H.P.: Sonar measurement of fetal crown-rump length as means of assessing maturity in first trimester of pregnancy. Brit. Med. J. 4:28, 1973.

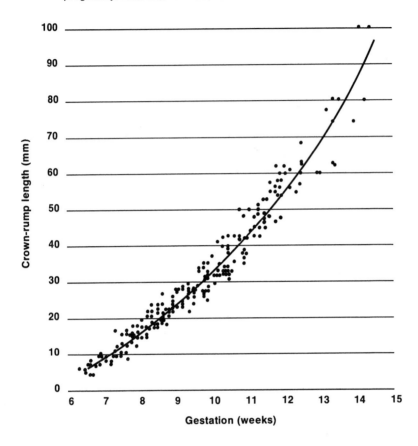

Figure 4

Crown-rump measurement as a determinant of fetal age. This
determination is a useful and sensitive indicator of gestational age.
In very early pregnancy some patience is required to obtain the
proper plane for measurement.

From Robinson, H.P., and Fleming J.E.E.: A critical evaluation of
sonar "crown-rump length" measurements. Brit. J. Obstet.
Gynaec. 82:702–710, 1975.

Menstrual Maturity (weeks + days)	CRL (mm) Mean	CRL (mm) 2 S.D.	Menstrual Maturity (weeks + days)	CRL (mm) Mean	CRL (mm) 2 S.D.
6 + 2	7.0	3.3	10 + 0	33.0	7.2
6 + 3	6.5	1.4	10 + 1	33.8	7.6
6 + 4	7.0	4.6	10 + 2	35.2	7.3
6 + 5	6.5	4.2	10 + 3	36.0	7.9
6 + 6	10.0	2.6	10 + 4	37.3	9.7
7 + 0	9.3	2.3	10 + 5	43.4	7.7
7 + 1	10.3	8.0	10 + 6	40.1	7.1
7 + 2	11.8	5.7	11 + 0	46.7	6.1
7 + 3	12.8	4.8	11 + 1	43.6	7.2
7 + 4	13.4	6.7	11 + 2	47.5	6.2
7 + 5	15.4	3.6	11 + 3	48.8	5.9
7 + 6	15.4	4.4	11 + 4	49.0	9.5
8 + 0	17.0	4.9	11 + 5	54.0	9.8
8 + 1	19.5	5.7	11 + 6	56.2	9.5
8 + 2	19.4	6.2	12 + 0	58.3	9.4
8 + 3	20.4	5.0	12 + 1	56.8	7.2
8 + 4	21.3	3.8	12 + 2	59.4	6.6
8 + 5	20.9	2.4	12 + 3	62.6	8.6
8 + 6	23.2	3.6	12 + 4	63.5	9.5
9 + 0	25.8	6.0	12 + 5	67.7	6.4
9 + 1	25.4	4.6	12 + 6	66.5	8.2
9 + 2	26.7	4.4	13 + 0	72.5	4.2
9 + 3	27.0	2.8	13 + 1	69.7	8.5
9 + 4	32.5	4.2	13 + 2	73.0	15.1
9 + 5	30.0	10.0	13 + 3	77.0	8.5
9 + 6	31.3	5.5	13 + 4	—	—
			13 + 5	—	—
			13 + 6	76.0	5.7
			14 + 0	79.6	7.8

Figure 5

Yale Nomogram for BPD Using Leading Edge to Leading Edge
Based on B-mode dots (Graticule)

cm	Weeks gestation	cm	Weeks gestation	cm	Weeks gestation
		4.2	18.9	6.9	28.1
		4.3	19.4	7.0	28.6
		4.4	19.4	7.1	29.1
		4.5	19.9	7.3	29.6
		4.6	20.4	7.4	30.0
		4.7	20.4	7.5	30.6
1.9	11.6	4.8	20.9	7.6	31.0
2.0	11.6	4.9	21.3	7.7	31.5
2.1	12.1	5.0	21.3	7.8	32.0
2.2	12.6	5.1	21.8	7.9	32.5
2.3	12.6	5.2	22.3	8.0	33.0
2.4	13.1	5.3	22.3	8.2	33.5
2.5	13.6	5.4	22.8	8.3	34.0
2.6	13.6	5.5	23.3	8.4	34.4
2.7	14.1	5.6	23.3	8.5	35.0
2.8	14.6	5.7	23.8	8.6	35.4
2.9	14.6	5.8	24.3	8.8	35.9
3.0	15.0	5.9	24.3	8.9	36.4
3.1	15.5	6.0	24.7	9.0*	36.9
3.2	15.5	6.1	25.2	9.1*	37.3
3.3	16.0	6.2	25.2	9.2*	37.8
3.4	16.5	6.3	25.7	9.3*	38.3
3.5	16.5	6.4	26.2	9.4*	38.8
3.6	17.0	6.5	26.2	9.6*	39.3
3.7	17.5	6.6	26.7	9.7*	39.8
3.8	17.9	6.7	27.2		
4.0	18.4	6.8	27.6		

* Indicates a fetus of 36 wks. or greater in a non-diabetic.

Figure 6

Nomogram for BPD Using Outer-to-Outer Edge

mm	Weeks gestation	mm	Weeks gestation	mm	Weeks gestation
23	13.1	49	19.5	75	29.0
24	13.3	50	19.8	76	29.4
25	13.5	51	20.1	77	29.9
26	13.7	52	20.4	78	30.4
27	13.9	53	20.7	79	30.8
28	14.1	54	21.0	80	31.3
29	14.3	55	21.4	81	31.8
30	14.6	56	21.7	82	32.3
31	14.8	57	22.0	83	32.8
32	15.0	58	22.4	84	33.3
33	15.3	59	22.7	85	33.8
34	15.5	60	23.1	86	34.3
35	15.7	61	23.4	87	34.8
36	16.0	62	23.8	88	35.4
37	16.2	63	24.1	89	35.9
38	16.5	64	24.5	90	36.5 *mature*
39	16.7	65	24.9	91	37.0
40	17.0	66	25.3	92	37.6
41	17.2	67	25.7	93	38.2
42	17.5	68	26.1	94	38.8
43	17.8	69	26.5	95	39.4
44	18.0	70	26.9	96	40.0
45	18.3	71	27.3	97	40.6
46	18.6	72	27.7	98	41.2
47	18.9	73	28.1	99	41.9
48	19.2	74	28.6	100	42.5

From Brown, R. E.: *Ultrasonography: Basic Principles and Clinical Application*. Warren H. Green, Inc., St. Louis.

Figure 7

Estimation of fetal weight and gestational age from biparietal diameter.

From Bartolucci, L.: Biparietal diameter of the skull and fetal weight in the second trimester: an allometric relationship. Am. J. Obstet. Gynec. 122:439–444, 1975.

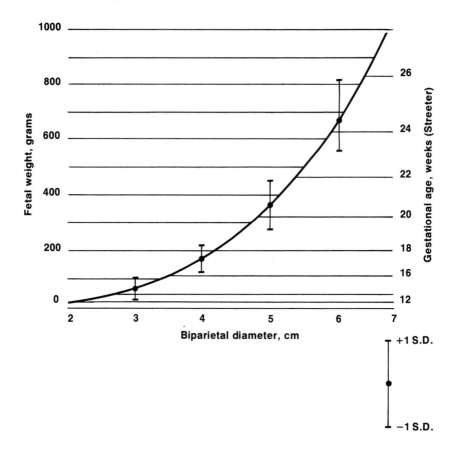

Figure 8

Transverse diameter of fetal trunk versus period of gestation.

From Garrett, W.J., and Robinson, D.E.: Assessment of fetal size and growth rate by ultrasonic echoscopy. Obstet. Gynec. 38:525–534, 1971.

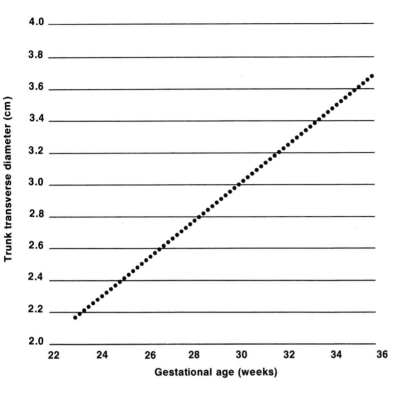

Figure 9

Cross section of an area of the fetal trunk versus period of gestation (weeks' amenorrhea).

From Garrett, W.J., and Robinson, D.E.: Assessment of fetal size and growth rate by ultrasonic echoscopy, Obstet. Gynec. 38:525–534, 1971.

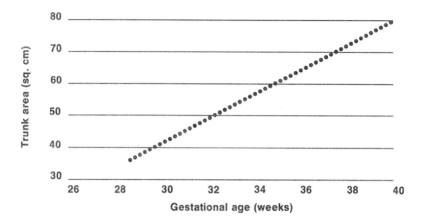

Figure 10

Cross section of an area of the fetal head versus period of gestation (weeks' amenorrhea).

From Garrett, W.J., and Robinson, D.E.: Assessment of fetal size and growth rate by ultrasonic echoscopy. Obstet. Gynec. 38:525–534, 1971.

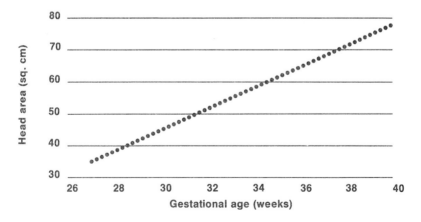

Figure 11

Relationship between fetal abdominal circumference
measurements from 21 to 40 cm. and birth weight centiles.

From Campbell, S., and Wilkin, D.: Ultrasonic measurement of fetal
abdomen circumference in the estimation of fetal weight. Brit. J.
Obstet. Gynaec. 82:689–697, 1975.

Abdominal Circumference (cm)	Estimated birth weight centiles (kg)				
	5*		50	95*	
21	0.78	(86.4)	0.90	1.04	(115.7)
22	0.90	(86.7)	1.03	1.19	(115.3)
23	1.03	(86.9)	1.18	1.36	(115.0)
24	1.17	(87.1)	1.34	1.54	(114.8)
25	1.32	(87.2)	1.51	1.73	(114.7)
26	1.47	(87.3)	1.69	1.94	(114.6)
27	1.64	(87.3)	1.88	2.15	(114.5)
28	1.81	(87.3)	2.09	2.38	(114.5)
29	1.99	(87.3)	2.28	2.61	(114.5)
30	2.17	(87.4)	2.49	2.85	(114.5)
31	2.35	(87.4)	2.69	3.08	(114.5)
32	2.53	(87.4)	2.90	3.32	(114.4)
33	2.71	(87.4)	3.10	3.55	(114.4)
34	2.88	(87.4)	3.29	3.76	(114.4)
35	3.03	(87.4)	3.47	3.97	(114.4)
36	3.18	(87.4)	3.64	4.16	(114.4)
37	3.31	(87.3)	3.79	4.33	(114.5)
38	3.42	(87.3)	3.92	4.49	(114.6)
39	3.51	(87.2)	4.02	4.61	(114.7)
40	3.57	(87.0)	4.10	4.72	(115.0)

*Figures in brackets represent the centile limit expressed as a percentage
of the median birth weight.

Figure 12

Abdominal circumference as a predictor of fetal weight. The circumference measurement is made at right angles to the fetal spine at the level of the umbilical vein (Chapter 6) with a map reader.

From Campbell, S., and Wilkin, D.: Ultrasonic measurement of fetal abdomen circumference in the estimation of fetal weight. Brit. J. Obstet. Gynaec. 82:689–697, 1975.

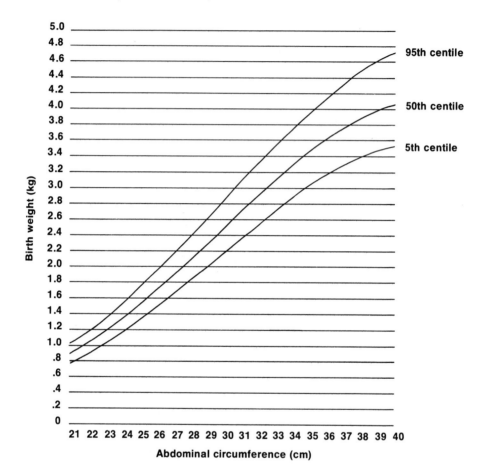

Figure 13

Fetal urine production rates at different times in gestation.

From Campbell, S., Wladimiroff, J.W., and Dewhurst, D.J.: The antenatal measurement of fetal urine production. J. Obstet. Gynec. 80:680–686, 1973.

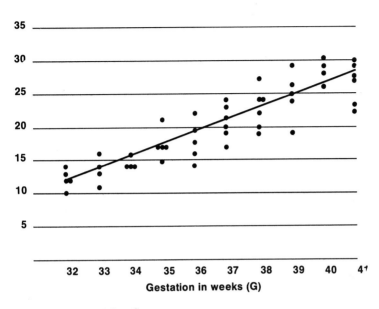

$\mu = -45.3 + 1.8 \times G$

$r = 0.8955$

Index